I0790465

God Said, "LIVE!"

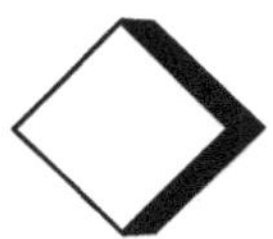

Harvey J. Morgan

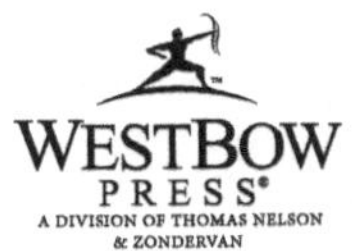

WestBow
PRESS®
A DIVISION OF THOMAS NELSON
& ZONDERVAN

WestBow Press books may be ordered through booksellers or by contacting:

WestBow Press
A Division of Thomas Nelson & Zondervan
1663 Liberty Drive
Bloomington, IN 47403
www.westbowpress.com
844-714-3454

Interior Image Credit: Harvey J. Morgan

Scripture taken from the King James Version of the Bible.

ISBN: 978-1-6642-4223-4 (sc)
ISBN: 978-1-6642-4224-1 (hc)
ISBN: 978-1-6642-4222-7 (e)

Library of Congress Control Number: 2021916047

Print information available on the last page.

WestBow Press rev. date: 12/08/2021

This book is dedicated to Brenda, my precious wife. Her stability has guided me through life. It is also dedicated to our four children—Becky, Mark, Terry, and Sherry (twins)—and their families. They have been our lives' greatest achievement.

FOREWORD

But the people that do know their God
shall be strong, and do exploits.
—Daniel 11:32

Most people go through life knowing only *about* God. They see creation and therefore know there must be a creator. They see radical change in the life of a new believer and recognize the work of a higher power. This kind of faith is much like seeing ripples on the water and knowing wind is a natural influence. But, rare as it may be, there are those who have gone beyond the veil and come away with a knowledge of God, which is as certain to them as 2+2 to a mathematician. Brother Morgan is such a man. Brother Junior Morgan knows his God.

Many years ago, I heard Brother Morgan talk about a man asking him whether he had ever had God "speak to him." "Yes," Brother Morgan replied. "In fact, He spoke to me this morning."

The man pressed, "How did you know He was speaking?"

With such deep emotion, I still feel his words nearly twenty years later, Brother Morgan replied, "I felt Him speak to me."

How does a man or woman get to this place of intimacy with God? What is the key? Where is the door? Devotion? Devotion is indeed an important component in the life of believers. I have witnessed firsthand the devotion of Brother Morgan. I have watched him wrestle in the altar for hours on end in prayer for those who were seeking spiritual freedom.

Is it sacrifice? Without question, sacrifice is expected of those who follow Christ. Paul made that abundantly clear in Romans 12:1. I was there when Brother Morgan was so weak from fasting that he required assistance to get to the pulpit. Perhaps suffering is the essential element? It was the mighty A.W. Tozer who said, "It is doubtful whether God can bless a man greatly until He has hurt him deeply." As you read the following pages, it will become clear that Brother Morgan knows much about suffering. Not only has he suffered physically and emotionally, but after decades of pastoral ministry, he knows well the wounds of a caring shepherd. But I believe the sure path to real relationship with God, the kind of relationship where you can deeply *feel* God speak to your heart, is paved with humility. And this, in my opinion, is Brother Morgan's foremost attribute. His eagerness to remain hidden behind the cross has allowed God to grant mighty miracles through his prayers.

The words you will read in the following chapters come from a man seeking to glorify God in every way he knows how. A man whose life isn't his own. A man who has been bought and belongs to another; and a man who would not have it any other way.

Dear reader, please understand that as you read this book, you are about to spend time with a man who knows His God.

Yours in Christ,
Jon Curtis Isaacs

ACKNOWLEDGMENTS

I wish to acknowledge Pineview Holiness Baptist Church, who stood with me through my sickness and recovery, and many church friends and community members, who sent encouraging messages to me and my family. Also, I wish to thank the sixth floor at Emory Winship Hospital and their excellent doctors, nurses, and other medical personnel, which included Dr. Arellano and her great staff. South Georgia Medicine, Dr. Don Roberts and Terry Morgan, PAC, provided a quick diagnosis of acute myeloid leukemia (AML), in conjunction with Dr. Shah and Tift Regional Oncology Center. In addition, our daughter, Becky, dedicated many hours compiling and reviewing the contents of this book.

CHAPTER 1

THE BEGINNING

God guides us through life in mysterious ways. We like to plan out how we think things should progress, but then we realize that we see only the circumstances that directly affect us. If we solely determined life's plans, we would choose the high road with the least amount of resistance every time. As Christians, though, we come face-to-face with times that shape and mold us into vessels God can work through. Those times of smooth sailing and storm-free days are easy to take for granted. We breathe in as though we are going to breathe and walk around like everything our feet touches will always be ours. This feeling of entitlement, where all feel like they have ownership over their lives and bodies, is often misplaced. After all, we Christians live surrendered lives.

We are guaranteed nothing, except that all things work for good to those who love God (Romans 8:28). No one knows when he or she is going to die or when he or she might be involved in a terrible accident. Similarly, we don't know whether the next moment might bring the news that could change our lives forever.

Such was the case for me. Before we begin, let me tell you a little about myself.

For my whole life, almost everyone has referred to me as "Junior" except when at school or in places where my official name had to be used. Honestly, my life was as happy and fulfilled as it could be. I was a loving son to my parents, a devoted husband to my wife, a caring father to my children, and a granddaddy. At the same time, I was a brother, uncle, friend, counselor, prayer warrior, pastor, barber and—a bit more humorously—a "tub doctor" by trade. I was a simple man with many hats living an incredibly happy life. For some reason, harsh things can seem magnified when there is so much good happening and smooth sailing on the horizon.

Things were going quite well when the bad news arrived.

Before we get more into that, let me elaborate more so you have an idea where I'm coming from and will understand more about my fight with calamity. I was born on September 11, 1949, to Clayton and Ada Morgan in Coffee County, Georgia. I had a sister, Doris, who was almost two years older than me. We were the typical brother and sister duo. We fought a lot and shared everything. We took each other's snacks and teased each other relentlessly.

When I was five, my family moved to Valdosta, Georgia, so my father could get a better job. He was a barber by trade, and he was also a deacon in our church, which required him to help run the church operations. My mom was our church secretary and a homemaker. Her church position required her to keep minutes (records) of business meetings and to be responsible for the church's financial operations. From the time since I was small, I have been part of what we call "the church."

People may call it naive, but there is something wonderfully mysterious about our world. When we think we begin to understand it, we come across something truly baffling but ultimately amazing. Maybe it's just my way of rationalizing the situation, but I believe that what happened to me played right into the mystery of the world. From the time I was a young child, I witnessed miracles and saw my parents, friends, and family worship the Lord through songs, prayer, and preaching. I am so glad now that I had the opportunity to grow up in the church age that I was raised in—to personally witness the miraculous and unexplainable.

I grew up attending Unity Church in Valdosta, which was part of a larger organization of churches, mainly in Georgia and Florida. The people in those churches were rural, country people who weren't wealthy, yet they valued family, faith, and freedom. They interpreted the Bible both literally and allegorically, which meant they applied it to their everyday lives. During those growing-up years, I wasn't necessarily fully interested in the actual church services. Like most boys and girls my age, I was more interested in spending time hanging out with my friends. Even in that part of my life, though, I understood what was going on in church services and in the world around me. Nevertheless, I didn't claim to be a Christian. I saw what was happening in the services, and I knew what my parents and friends were doing in their worship, but I didn't commit myself to do the same at a young age.

All I knew was that when I did become a Christian, I wanted to have as dedicated and faithful experiences as the people I had witnessed in my family, and this included serving a powerful God. If God brought you to it, He will bring you through it (as He did for the children of Israel). These churches believed in the saving power of the blood of Jesus, as described in John 3:16. "For God so loved the world, that He gave his only begotten Son, that whosoever believeth in him should not perish, but have everlasting life." They also believed that with His stripes, we are healed (Isaiah 53:5). Church wasn't just something they had to attend on a Sunday morning. Instead, church was a daily walk of submission to the will and purpose of God. We usually gathered for Sunday morning, Sunday evening, and a midweek service. Also there was usually Sunday school an hour before the morning service and church revival at least four times a year. Revival times were where people were fervently stirred to rededicate their lives to Christ if they had become slack and prayed for lost people in their communities to come to know the Lord. Their lives inspired me to search for that "highway of Holiness" Isaiah talked about in Isaiah 35:8. I admired how they lived, worshipped, and praised God, and I wanted to join them.

I feel I am truly blessed by God to have such a foundation of faith.

The age of seventeen was a turning point in my life. There was such a vivid memory for me that I still remember the exact date: October 18, 1966. On that day, I decided that I would dedicate my entire life to the Lord; thus, I was "born again," according to John 3:16. My life was transformed by the power of the blood of Jesus, and several changes were made. For instance, I was somewhat mischievous back then, like most kids in their teens. As somewhat of a prankster, I spent time with my buddies, who were like me: a troublemaker. When I became a new creature in Christ, the old things passed away, and my life changed for the better. My friends could tell my life was different now.

After my conversion to Christ, I was usually quiet in a crowd. I didn't like being the center of attention in most cases. My nature is still somewhat shy in that I don't like to be in the spotlight. Several months after my born-again experience, I understood that my simple church attendance wasn't enough for me to live a fully consecrated life. I wasn't interested in fulfilling some form of formality. Instead, I felt a yearning inside me to do more.

Thus, in April 1967, I felt the call to preach the gospel. I wanted to carry the good message of the gospel of Jesus Christ to the world, who didn't know Him as their personal Savior. I began to reach out to people to let them know the Lord would like to be their personal guide through life. I found that many people will initially reject the call of God to become His child, but when calamity strikes, they are often found trying to find God. My message is for them to seek the Lord while He is near. It is wonderful to have Him already as your Lord before the time of trouble comes.

In November 1967, I met Brenda Watson from Nashville, Georgia, and we married in 1968. Little did she know that she would become part of a ministry team. Wherever I went, she would follow. In 1969 and 1970, I pastored my first church in Iron City, Georgia. My wife and I were itinerant pastors, traveling 102 miles one way, two Sundays a month. Sometimes crowds were small, but that fact didn't discourage us, and we remained faithful.

Most of my experience in preaching and pastoring was birthed at this church. On Sundays, we went home with someone from the church for lunch and remain there until the night's service. After the evening service, we drove back to Valdosta to start the workweek again early Monday morning.

As time went on, I pastored several small country churches. I preached revivals, youth camps, and camp meetings. I also conducted funerals and weddings, and my family expanded to include our first daughter, Becky; a son, Mark; and twins: a boy and a girl, Terry and Sherry.

Besides all the pastoral duties I attended, I also went on mission trips to Trinidad and Costa Rica. I preached in brush arbor meetings, outdoor tent meetings, and in-home prayer services.

In 1976, when the twins were about six weeks old, a great tragedy happened to me. Though many considered it to be an expected part of life, it was very difficult for me to bear as I watched my mother die from lymphoma. This was a devastating time, which tried the foundations of my faith.

My parents had lived next door to us for many years. My mother was our babysitter when my wife went to college and later began teaching. The fact that she died broke my heart, even though I knew it was what God intended. Yet it still caused me much grief. I watched my mother suffer, but I made peace with the fact that God's will must be done, no matter what the circumstances. There are a lot of times in life when a person just doesn't understand the chaos around him or her. However, in these times, he or she must trust God because even in the chaos, there is order. It might not be noticeably clear, but it is always right there. As time went on and

I healed from the wound of my mother's passing, I continued my pastorate.

In 1992, we began our longest pastorate in Moultrie, Georgia, at Liberty Faith Holiness Church. We went there as a "fill-in" pastor. We enjoyed the worship services there immensely, and the people were friendly and genuine. They called us to be their pastor, and I felt that this was a divine appointment. I humbly accepted the call to be their pastor. Consequently, the church continued to grow by country church standards. As time continued, I felt the need to start a Christian school for my church children and children in the surrounding community. My desire was for the youth to focus on God's direction as well as to pay attention to academia. After acquiring donations and meeting with the church committee, we started a Christian school. Since then, it has been a stable influence in the community, and it just completed its twenty-sixth year.

Our church also worked to start a local grocery assistance program. We helped seven hundred people per month with household groceries, accepting donations to this program for its upkeep. Liberty Faith also maintained a local radio program every Sunday afternoon, where our sole purpose was to reach as many people with the gospel as we could. The radio program was live, and many people attended and participated in it. Sometimes the crowd filled the radio station. It was a great tradition the community enjoyed for years. For us, church itself has always been active—more than just what happens inside the four walls on Sunday.

Everyone who was part of our church wanted to be part of getting the message of the gospel out to the local area. They wanted people to know the church loved them as Jesus did. They told the message of how one could come to Jesus and start life anew. Daily, I encountered many people who were searching for divine guidance. Consequently, I felt the need for a significant revival in our area. I wanted our children and youth in the church to see and experience an old-fashioned Holy Ghost revival like days of old. To pursue this, several of us from the church banded together with much self-sacrifice, fasting meals for several consecutive days.

During that time, my faith and experience with the Lord grew more profoundly as our church and many visitors saw and experienced many divine healings and deliverances. People attended from far and near. The Lord blessed in miraculous ways. Many people were born again. We had revival church services for eight weeks, but the spirit of revival continued for several years. Based on the promises in God's Word, I knew He would hear and answer prayers and that He would do abundantly more than we could think or ask. The highlight of my ministry was that I baptized one hundred people during one year after the great revival that spanned serval weeks. Seeing the birth of a strong youth group, witnessing the growth of their roots of faith, and participating in spiritually strong revival established my ministry and created the desire to maintain a strong outreach to the lost world for Christ.

Through life's ups and downs of raising children and counseling other people in churches I had pastored, I continued to believe God in all situations. I am blessed to say all our children became Christians at an early age, between the ages of seven and thirteen. They had seen their parents remain faithful and determined in every circumstance that came from life. They also completed college degrees and entered the professional world, still maintaining their Christian faith. Even though all of them are grown and married, they have reared their children in active churches and continue to participate in regular worship services and Christian outreach activities until this present day.

After seventeen years, I resigned the pastorate at Liberty Faith to evangelize, preaching revivals and weekend services in various states. After three years, I began filling in at Pineview Holiness Baptist Church in Tifton, Georgia, because they were without a pastor. After preaching for them for several weekends, they asked me to become their full-time pastor. Since I trust God with my life,

I allowed Him to lead me, even though I was reaching the elder pastor status of life.

Sometimes it seems that the faith of people who have lived their lives in pursuit of God is tested by the greatest of difficulties. The greatest challenge for me came in the form of a diagnosis. In November or December of 2013, the Lord revealed that He would give Pineview a mighty miracle for a testimony. At the end of January 2014, while preaching a revival meeting in Wilson, North Carolina, I noticed a physical weakness in my body. I finished the revival, went home, and scheduled a family meal to have all my children and grandchildren around me. I let them know that something was very wrong. However, I attempted to continue to preach and fulfill my pastoring duties.

After our family gathering on Saturday, February 1, 2014, I went for bloodwork the following Monday, as ordered by our son Terry, who is a physician's assistant. The report came back that my blood counts weren't normal. Upon the insistence of doctors, I was admitted to a local hospital because of my compromised immune system. I also had a bone marrow test, which Dr. Shah ordered from the oncology center in Tifton. The bone marrow test came back positive for a form of leukemia, with the most likely diagnosis as acute myeloid leukemia (AML). I stayed quarantined in the hospital at Tifton until Thursday afternoon so appointments could be made for a possible trip to Emory Hospital in Atlanta. Through the weekend, we stayed at home, seeing only close family members due to my weakened immune system and not knowing what we were possibly facing over the weeks and months ahead.

After watching my mother suffer with lymphoma, I knew this diagnosis would be life changing. My heart quaked within me, and I could see fear and worry start to invade my family circle. The furtive looks, the quiet whispers, the flowing tears—what in the world would we do now? Then I saw the shoulders square back, the heads bow down, and the lips move in prayer, resolving to *still* trust Him, who has always been in control.

CHAPTER 2

DIAGNOSIS (DAYS 1–6)

Day 1

Monday, February 10, started out as a regular day. Both my wife, Brenda, and I were running about our normal routines. She left to teach her college classes at Valdosta State University, while I was waiting at home. I was somewhat anxious while sitting around and waiting for a call from the doctor's office. At approximately 8:30 a.m., the phone rang. This may seem early to some people, but I get an early start to my day, so this isn't too early for phone calls at our house. They told me I had to report to Emory University Hospital by 2 p.m.

I immediately called Terry and Mark to devise a plan for getting to Atlanta, which is a four-hour trip. Meanwhile, Terry tried calling Brenda so she would know what was transpiring. Obviously, things began going wrong right from the start. Brenda had left her phone at home that day. However, we couldn't leave without Terry talking to Brenda, so we had to figure out another way.

We were finally able to contact the Math Department at the university to get a message to Brenda, asking her to call home at her earliest convenience. He also called his sisters, Becky and Sherry, so they could let their families know. With his extensive medical background and involvement in the bloodwork and treatment thus far, he provided all the information he was aware of up until this point. I'm not going to lie; things didn't look good. All the family members were terribly upset upon hearing the news.

The next steps had been laid out for us: get to Atlanta to determine where to go from there. I started packing my pajamas and struggled to get into the shower since I was feeling quite weak. While making my way out of the bathtub after getting done with my shower, I felt as if the Lord were reaching out to me. *Remember Ezekiel 16:6. You're going to need it in the next few weeks.* I was familiar with the verse of scripture, which reads, "And when I passed by thee and saw thee polluted in thine own blood, I said unto thee when thou wast in thy blood, Live: yea, I said unto thee when thou wast in thy blood, Live." Completely shaken by my reality, I started to find some sort of solace in this experience. Having our Lord reach out to me gave me peace. It reminded me that while not everything is in our control, I believe God has supreme authority over everything.

I got out of the shower to find that Mark had arrived at the house, with Becky, Sherry, and Silas (my son-in-law who is better known as Doodle Bug) not far behind. They were able to contact Brenda at VSU, and she also arrived shortly. In our family discussion, we determined that I would go on to Emory with Mark and Terry. The rest of the family members who were able to travel would do so within a few hours.

We had to be at the doctor's office by 2 p.m. Mark and I left quickly from the family meeting after discussing the essential things on our way to pick up Terry. After getting on the road to Atlanta, we discussed the seriousness of the disease. We talked about what to do if the prognosis was hopeless or terminal. The discussion was deeper than it seems. It touched all my heartstrings. I wasn't sure how I should feel. I couldn't tell whether it was anxiety, fear, the yearning to be cured, or a bit of everything combined. Nonetheless,

I contributed to the conversation after putting in immense efforts to suppress the thoughts of calamity creeping into my brain.

I was worried sick, thinking, *Who will look after the estate and the property holdings?* I specified that taking care of Mom and her things was the most significant topic for me. The trip was long and grueling with unanswered questions in everyone's minds—both spoken and unspoken. I knew God was with us, but we wondered where the journey would lead. Most of the way, I found that I was talking to myself quite a lot. The thought of God being with me was the only thing that provided me satisfaction in this chaos. My life was so uncertain at this point that I wasn't sure about anything in it. However, one thing remained certain—God wouldn't leave me. So, as long as I reached out to Him, He would always reach out to me. Ah, doesn't that thought instantly calm you down?

We arrived at the Winship Emory Cancer Institute to meet with Dr. Martha Arellano and determine our next steps in dealing with this terminal disease. We came to this specific treatment center based on the referral of a local oncologist, Dr. Apurva Shah. After reviewing the medical information, Dr. Arellano gave orders for me to be admitted into Emory University Hospital.

Shortly after our arrival, I was admitted and assigned to room E605. Over the next several days, this room became home for me. The idea of a hospital room being a place where I would spend the most time wasn't a concept with which I was familiar. Is anyone really, though? However, when the going gets tough, you must get tougher.

I didn't have a choice. So crying about it would only make the situation all the worse. But let's be honest. The room was quite dull. The view from the window left me staring at part of the hospital roof, with buildings crammed together in the busy metropolitan area. It is much different from the calm countryside view from home—one of the many changes I had to become accustomed to. I didn't know how much time I would have to spend in the busy city, so I tried to be as receptive as I could to all these changes.

Inside my private room, there was a hospital bed; a long couch, which would fold down and make a very hard bed; and an upright chair, which filled one corner. The room also had a nightstand and a wall of lights, which allowed the medical personnel to easily see reports when they came in to conduct their examinations. Several plugs were scattered around. The wall across from the bed held a small whiteboard, where the hospital staff wrote the names of those who would be responsible for my care, based on their shifts. I also had a sink with some counter space. The room also had a bathroom, which included a shower area and toilet. I hope I was able to provide a vivid picture of my home. It is, in fact, something I had very carefully observed. I tried to distract myself using the lights placed there. I looked at them as something that illuminated the oh-so-dull room.

Nonetheless, the room was quite institutionalized but part of the package deal. I thought I would be stuck in that room all by myself, but instantly, my room was crawling with people coming and going. They introduced themselves as techs, nurses, orderlies, housekeepers, and others in various roles. Usually, the thought of hospital staff isn't one that comes across as a calm one. However, to my surprise, these very people became my closest pillars—the pillars who provided me with the hope, warmth, and encouragement I needed during those days. Maybe God sent me to this certain hospital for a reason. He knew the staff there would be quite welcoming and that my friends were the silver lining I needed to make it through these tough times.

I didn't let my sickness stop me from doing what I loved. The staff was quite respectful of me and even more so when they found out I was a preacher and a pastor. Whenever I had an opportunity, I shared the gospel with them, and all of them listened respectfully.

While I was getting settled in my room, Brenda and the other family members arrived. All of them were welcomed after dealing with plans to cover their responsibilities back home. These plans ranged from continuing their jobs, getting classes covered, making other job arrangements, and determining childcare for some of the grandchildren. Our family had never faced a crisis such as this. But one thing we did know was that no one would fight this battle alone. We would face it together as a family.

It's during times like these that you get to know who is there for you and who isn't. I'm very thankful to God, for He is the One who bestowed on me this blessing of being born into such a family. Even during a calamity, there were things I was thankful for. In fact, my disease made me see greater things in life that exist, but we often don't acknowledge them. At that point in time, I realized God had been so kind to me.

Not knowing how long or what the next few days or weeks would bring, Mark started a blog so we could connect with friends and family and keep them updated with our progress. Close family friends, my children's work friends, social media acquaintances, parishioners from the various churches I pastored, and community members started expressing concerns and sending messages of prayers for us. This blog acted as a strengthening factor for me. I continued to receive incoming messages, which gave me encouragement and reminded me of the compassion of my people while instilling warmth inside me. At the same time, I wanted people to have a way to stay updated with the news. There was also a unique option Mark added to the blog. In any case of emergency from either end (the posting and the reader end), there was a "remind" notification alert. Through this, the family could post prayer requests for the public in times of need and provide updates, for that matter.

God is always there to answer our prayers. The thought of so many people coming together and praying for me gave me great comforting feelings. But this time my friends were different. They were calmer and more positive. The idea of so many people praying to God for me kept me from being discouraged and gave me hope for a better future.

Some more family members made it to the hospital to see my new accommodations. They were also keen to meet with the team of doctors, who would confirm my diagnosis and present my treatment options.

Day 2

This day presented what would become our motto: hurry up and wait. Some medical staff would come in and say, "Today, the doctor has ordered a certain test. They will come and take you to a specific lab." Thinking the test could happen any minute, we constantly watched the door and anxiously waited for the next staff member to come in and for the process to begin. There was always a flurry of activity, with staff coming and going, getting blood drawn every few hours, and records being maintained. But there was this constant waiting for what would be next.

All my medical records from Tift Regional Medical Center (now called Southwell Health) were added to my file at Emory, and the doctors' team worked to confirm my diagnosis. I could see that my family members would also be feeling the same thing as me. Sometimes I felt as if they were more concerned than I was. Perhaps the thought of losing a family member is more severe to the human heart than we can comprehend.

Dr. Arellano met with the family members, who were able to meet around my hospital bed, and she used the room's whiteboard to present us with the treatment options for my diagnosis: acute myeloid leukemia (AML). She presented us with three different treatment options if the diagnosis was indeed correct. Two of these treatments involved experimental drugs in addition to standard therapy. If I didn't agree to treatment, the doctor said I had less than two months to live. On the other hand, if I decided to undergo this excruciating treatment, I needed to be wary of the fact that there was only a 5 percent recovery chance.

When the doctor asked me what I wanted to do, I told her I wasn't afraid to die. Honestly speaking, I didn't shiver once while saying this statement. The words were truly what I felt from the inside. I had served the Lord for forty-six years in preparation for this time—my time to meet the Lord. I told the doctor that if I died, I was confident in knowing I was on my way to meet my Lord. The doctor looked at me with a questioning look as I shared my thoughts with her, but I was serious.

My children were in shock and disbelief, not knowing which option would be best. The doctor said she would let us all discuss it and that she would be back later. I asked my wife and all my children to leave E605 while I prayed alone to determine what to do. I knew only God could provide me with the right answer. He has always looked after me, and even during such times, I knew He would reach out to me.

My family went down to the hospital chapel to pray and have their own discussion. At the time, I didn't know Terry had told them that if I went home without this treatment, it would be a terribly painful death. I wish they had been unaware of this fact. Then maybe if I decided not to go ahead with the treatment, it wouldn't hurt them so much. They all prayed together in the chapel, and I prayed in the hospital room. When they came back to the room, they found my Bible opened to Ezekiel 16:6, with teardrops on the pages, but I wasn't there.

They told me later that they weren't sure whether I had left or where exactly I was. One of the nurses told them I had been taken to have a procedure. I had to have an "echo" (echocardiogram) done to see whether my heart was strong enough for the impending treatment. The results showed that my heart was essentially normal. The family cried together, knowing that a battle loomed on the horizon. But we said this: "What shall we then say to these things? If God be for us, who can be against us?" (Romans 8:31).

As the day wore on, we continued to discuss the treatment options. I had watched my mother suffer from the treatment for lymphoma, and I didn't want to experience that same discomfort and pain. However, I wanted to be submissive to the Lord. He promised to be with me in every situation, no matter what I faced. I knew that even if things were hard, I had faith that He would see me through. I remembered the promise described in Ezekiel 16:6. When God says, "Live," there really is no choice but to live, whatever that encompasses. It's not like I was choosing to die, but instead, the idea of death didn't scare me. So opting not to take the treatment was something I was okay with. However, I knew my family would be quite hurt if I didn't do all I could to remain here.

According to weather reports, an ice storm would be moving in soon, and many family members had to return home. Meanwhile, Mark and Terry remained with me at the hospital. We shared a tearful goodbye, with none of us sure of what the next few days would bring. As I was hugging my family members goodbye, I could feel my heart sink. With each hug, the sinking feeling got deeper and deeper. Along with the goodbyes, I thought this was as worse as it could get until I moved onto my next hug. The whole process was beautiful yet so dreadful for me.

Day 3

On Wednesday, our third day at Emory, the ice storm outside prevented the research team from being present. This led to a delay, and the decisions on the treatment couldn't be finalized. I had to spend the majority of the morning in the Interventional Radiology Department getting a PICC line, a more permanent IV line where the chemotherapy could be given and blood could be drawn without having to stick a needle in me every time. I was already so weak, both physically and mentally, yet one thing remained constant. I didn't stop trusting God for a miracle. After all, He said, "Live." I knew I had to do whatever it took to live.

Whatever I couldn't do, I knew He could. We still debated and prayed about which method to choose.

After the consistent blood draws that reflected the white blood cell counts, the medical team added a couple of medications to help control them. As best as we knew, induction chemotherapy would begin in the next two to four days. While I slept, Mark and Terry explored the university hospital and the surrounding eating areas. They were limited in what they could do due to the ice storm and its effects on the area. I knew I was the patient here, but I couldn't help feeling bad for Mark and Terry. I felt as if I were causing added pain to the people I loved. Everyone was emotionally exhausted, and now I felt so bad to see those two draining themselves physically due to the restless stays at the hospital.

Day 4

Thursday showed us more of what the ice storm of 2014 was known for: shutting down travel and anything unnecessary in an area not accustomed to snow and layers of ice. This meant nobody could leave or, for that matter, come to visit me at the hospital.

We spent this day mostly waiting (remember, hurry up and wait). The research team with the trial drug treatments were still unable to get together to discuss and confirm the experimental trials. I felt like I was just getting ready—not sure what I was getting ready for—and just preparing. I walked around the wing on the sixth floor, meeting and greeting others, who were also stranded at the hospital, either for treatments or for visiting family members on the wing.

Never in my life had I felt more lost. I didn't know what I was preparing myself for. Any step I took toward a potential treatment only led me to take further steps in the opposite direction because no decision could yet be made. So here I was: just strolling about the hospital. There is an extremely strict protocol for visitors on this floor, and many precautions were made to protect the patients. The boys and I walked twenty-five laps around the wing, knowing that twenty-one laps made one mile. I had permission to be out of my room if I stayed on the wing on the sixth floor. I wasn't officially a prisoner to my disease, and I wasn't going to become one either.

I had some tough moments on this day, realizing that it would be four to six weeks at the earliest before I could see my home in rural South Georgia. This realization struck me hard. Before, I was clueless as to how long it would take. However, now that I had some numbers to put to this whole situation, oddly enough, everything started to become more real. An interesting concept the boys introduced to me to was the ability to "FaceTime" with the other children, who couldn't be here because of the storm, along with their spouses, grandchildren, and of course, my wife.

They all loved to make silly faces and use filters to take screenshots; I didn't realize until later how silly they sometimes made me look. These little connections to home and family meant the world to me. I wished I could be there with them, but I knew they were praying for me, and I knew they wanted the best for our family. These were the people I would count on the most (along with my church family) to help win this battle against my sickness. Even though I couldn't be in their physical presence, they were giving me the best gift of all—the gift of prayer. Prayer is something I believe in very deeply. It is something I have advocated all my life. Therefore, knowing my loved ones were there for me through prayers was a different comfort.

Day 5

Activity on Friday started at around 7 a.m. Nausea prevented me from eating much breakfast, but IV medication really helped after about twenty minutes. Mark and Terry decided to read me some of the comments and encouraging messages from visitors who were appearing on the blog. All the words from our friends, neighbors, and extended family members were so uplifting and encouraging. Dr. Arellano and the medical team were able to visit, and they determined that chemo could be started the next Monday.

The rest remained normal. Following my usual routine in the hospital, there were constant temperature checks, blood draws, blood pressure checks, and other monitoring being done. I had to finish some other tests today to complete the preparation for the induction chemo. We had another bone marrow biopsy completed, and we would love to be able to stand before the medical team and tell them two words: "But God." But if we had to walk this journey, it was surely a comfort to know God would walk it with us, along with the innumerable saints, who had pledged their prayers and thoughts. It became a daily ritual for whoever stayed with me at the hospital to read the blog comments at the end of each day and any time we felt like we needed to beat back the oppression or depression that tried to find its way into E605.

I knew God was helping me through these posted comments. He sent me constant support by showing how many people loved me during my time of need. I knew I had people who were there for me. "We are troubled on every side, yet not distressed; we are perplexed, but not in despair" (2 Corinthians 4:8). We knew our God had an army of saints who were praying on our behalf, and we could feel the strength of each prayer being sent for us. We were still holding on to Ezekiel 16:6. I don't think I will ever be able to let go of this verse. It's just one of those things ingrained inside me, something that is part of me. And how can one let go of one of his or her parts? For it is a piece that makes the whole possible.

Day 6

On Saturday, February 15, I awoke to agonizing pain radiating around my left side, which was probably due to the bone marrow biopsy performed yesterday. I could barely stand. My body curled itself, and my jaws clenched due to the excruciating pain running throughout my system. I really couldn't tell whether it was my insides that were hurting or my outer body. Dr. Arellano thought a nerve could have been hit during the procedure, which can sometimes happen. I had to have medication to control this pain, which resulted in severe waves of nausea and dry heaving.

My family did their best to hold pans for my nausea and wipe my forehead. This experience only made me realize there were many more days of this ahead—more days of being sick, more days of having to have someone help me in the bed or out of bed or not be able to leave the bed at all. I knew God wouldn't put more on me than I could bear, and even though I was moving slowly today, I was still moving. A fellow pastor came by to bring me encouraging words, saying the race didn't go to the fast or to the swift but to the one who endured to the end.

Reminders that triggered the promises of God were the ones that got me by. Every time I felt like my body was giving up, I reminded myself that God wouldn't burden me more than I can bear. He wouldn't, absolutely *not*, burden me more than I could bear. I said this truth aloud thrice, and it still hit me like a fresh, new thought. It rejuvenated me.

Just as the pain and discomfort presented themselves, the blessings started showing up, too. For indeed, God only puts His best through the pain, for pain has hidden blessings that come with it. Visitors from different churches came, even people from hundreds of miles away. One group of young people from Liberty Faith Holiness Church rented a bus together and came to personally let me know they were fighting with me. One of the members of the group had started a personal fast and wouldn't eat until I went home. Her fast lasted forty days. While they were here, they sang worship songs and prayed, and we were greatly encouraged. (Here is a link to the YouTube video of that time: https://youtu.be/icKlFWO_56s.) Several of the parishioners from Pineview Holiness

Baptist Church also came to express to me that victory was indeed going to be won.

The idea that I had touched so many lives was unbelievable. It made me forget the pain I was going through. Sometimes a loss seems great, but just when you think you've hit the darkest hour, God comes with the ray of light. I truly experienced that the gain, indeed, is much more than the loss we face in our lives. At every single point, moment, and fleeting second, we have something to be thankful for. I had something to be thankful for as well. When push comes to shove, nothing feels better than feeling the presence of God and holding onto the everlasting bond that exists between the two of you.

Looking back over the pictures and recalling that day, I can see that a life of service can impact many people of all ages, even for years to come. If God said, "Live," I must not be finished. It is never too late to hope for a miracle. I learned that you need to ask God, for He will always answer your prayers, no matter how impossible they may seem. I held onto God, and He held onto me. I wouldn't have made it out if my bond hadn't existed with Him. It's because of this one sacred and oh-so-personal relationship that everything in my life has been so blessed. Be it my family or those very people who came out in my support; everything in my life, I owe to God.

Many years ago, I preached a message about the little Shunamite woman. With more trouble in her life than she could fathom, she was asked, "How is it with thee?" Her response was felt by everyone present that Saturday on the sixth floor of Emory University Hospital in room E605, and it is still my response ... *It is well!* (2 Kings 4:26).

CHAPTER 3

DIFFICULT DAYS AHEAD (DAYS 7–11)

Day 7

When I woke up on the seventh day, the pain from the previous day was gone, but a new, unexpected painful problem developed overnight. I now had severe swelling and pain in my left knee. It was also unbelievably sensitive. It took two grown men to get me to my feet, but then I began to collapse because of the pain. It seemed that my joint was septic. From no warning to just a sudden septic joint! Then simultaneously, my temperature spiked to 103.8. Immediate activity increased in and out of room E605, with medical staff and nurses and doctors moving in and out. They were getting blood cultures and bringing IV broad spectrum antibiotics, steroids, and pain meds. With this increase in medications came the onset of more nausea and dry heaves.

At that point, I was miserable, and there seemed to be nothing working to bring me out of the physical, miserable state. The increased temperature along with the pain made me long for the land of no pain and no trouble. When I started talking about my home in heaven, where there would be no pain or suffering, my children grew quiet. I told them I had been preparing to make that crossing for over forty years and that I wasn't afraid. They watched me with tears in their eyes, and then they decided to read me some of the comments from the website to encourage me and assure me that people were thinking about me and praying for me.

We had comments from other states, where a friend said, "Praying and believing with you guys for a miracle!" Young men from the church I had previously pastored sent words like, "We have been praying for you. Believing God for another miracle … the God that healed you of migraine headaches (instantly) is the same God that can heal you now! Looking for that miracle. Remember Isaiah 54:17. 'No weapon that is formed against thee shall prosper.' We Love You" (Dain & Rachael Croft). Another message said, "God said, 'Let the weak say, I am strong' (Joel 3:10)—This was reminded to us, and we believe God will do a great work!" (Cliff Howard). Children's coworkers and people from the community said, "Praying for strength and patience in the days ahead! Keep us posted as we all 'pray him back' home" (Denise Tucker).

Knowing people had taken time out of their schedules and busy days to send me words of encouragement really meant a lot to me and my family. My family watched as my strength was renewed and watched as "the weak became strong." It was amazing to see the power of the Word of God.

I was able to sleep some in the afternoon, and my children have told me that while I was sleeping, I raised my hand and pointed, like I do when preaching, and that I called someone's name. It was a name they all knew but one we hadn't really talked about in a while. This person was someone we all dearly loved, someone who once had a closer walk with his heavenly Father. Even in my sleep, they said I was reaching for a lost soul. It has been my life's work to reach for the lost, to cry to this world, that Jesus saves, and still be a voice crying in the wilderness. In my subconscious state, I was reaching out for the eternal soul of someone in a backslidden condition. The cry of my heart was still to reach the lost, to shout as loudly as I could, "Don't wait too late!"

The children worked out a rotation so two members of the family could stay with me at the hospital, while others went back to their jobs and families. Then on the weekends, the family gathered at the hospital to be together with me, to let me know I wasn't alone. They each stayed approximately three nights; then new family members came in. They had to be extremely cautious, and if any of them were sick, they had to trade so I wouldn't be exposed to their sickness.

The grandchildren came up with their families on the weekend and stayed on the hospital floor near the sixth floor in a waiting room. If I was feeling well enough, the doctors allowed me to roll down to the waiting room, wearing a mask so I could visit with them for a few minutes. They often had songs to share just to let me know they loved me and were ready for me to get back home so I could make them some homemade ice cream. Here is a link to one of the videos when they came to sing: https://www.youtube.com/watch?v=YQ1LnVSbCqM.

As day 7 wound to an end, they told me I referred to what they call a "Claytonisn." A Claytonism is something my father, Clayton Morgan, would say. "This has been the biggest hurry-up, do-nothing day!" is what I said, referring to the wonderful nursing staff, who rushed around doing things I couldn't see. Of course, the staff had many other patients and other documentation processes they had to tend to, but it felt to me at the time like they were rushing around, but I couldn't see the completion of their tasks. They all just laughed at me, but we all thanked God for His mercy and still knew something special was taking place. From that moment on, my family still declared, "We believe!" So "fear thou not; for I am with thee: be not dismayed; for I am thy God: I will strengthen thee; yea, I will help thee; yea, I will uphold thee with the right hand of my righteousness" (Isaiah 41:10).

Day 8

Days at the hospital sometimes blended into the night, with such an early start as they usually had. Blood draws were ever so many hours, and then results came in early. My overall white blood cell count was normal on day eight, and they were able to stop some of the medications that could have been contributing to my nausea. A rheumatologist who aspirated some fluid from my left knee to do further testing was one of the many doctors we saw today. Since the last bone marrow biopsy results were still pending, the oncologist further discussed the treatment. We were still praying for favorable results, along with hundreds of people who had contacted us on the blog and website.

All through the day, I heard stories of how our website and blog were touching people. They just wanted to read the story of my journey, but they ended up encouraged and strengthened. My children commented that this was a reminder to them of how I have lived my life. According to my children, "Daddy has been known as both a humble servant and as a warrior of faith—and this journey will be no different. The aches and pains, the raging fevers, and the helplessness reveal and show humility and suffering, while at the same time they require him to fight against those things that destroy peace, comfort, and normal body functions."

I didn't know that my children were saying such things about me, but they wanted me to include that in my description of these dark days. My family clung to the promise that we "are fearfully and wonderfully made" (Psalm 139:14). Visitors reminded us that God knows how to fix this creation; we just have to trust that He knows what is best for us. Other visitors today came carrying spiritual banners with "Survivor" as their testimonies, having survived this fight already and emerging victorious through the grace of God.

I have fought many battles during this Christian journey, but I have never faced one quite like this. However, I am more determined than ever to "live," according to the directive from

Ezekiel 16:6. No matter what, I believe God! Even in this bed of affliction, I wanted my children to know that as an old soldier of the cross, I had full confidence to say, "The battle is not mine" and "Rejoice not against me, O mine enemy: when I fall, I shall arise" (Micah 7:8). This battle was the most difficult trial we, the family, had faced, yet it was proving to be the most inspirational. How could something be so terrible and yet so great? How could it be both crushing and incredibly uplifting? How could it cause tears of immense pain and tears of joy? One of the goals of raising my children in Christian service was to show them that the flesh was weak but not the spirit. My flesh called this situation terrible, crushing, and painful; but our spirits called it inspirational, great, and uplifting. Our spirits saw this situation for what it really was to the believer—a chance for our God to move mightily, an instance where people must say, "Brother, that was God!"

I'm still amazed by the vast array of comments from blog readers, people who have meant so much to our family over the years and from new friends we have made since being at Emory. I had overwhelming support from churches, from the workplaces of my children, and from individuals. According to the blog, I had people who were continually fasting and praying on my behalf and on the behalf of my family, who were traveling from home to Atlanta during the week and on weekends to spend time up there with me.

I'm just a two-by-four preacher, just a plug (that's another Claytonism, according to my family). According to my son Mark, that is the reason so many people reached out to me. "He has been that 'plug' which stood in the gap to prevent souls from being carried downstream to destruction," Mark further explained. "Now, in this great battle, we, along with our friends and family, are cheering him on. We can't run this race for him, but we can sure run it with him." Another family member reported that while sleeping, I said, "I might be able to find me a place to shout!" To my family that meant victory was coming. And when it fully arrived, we were going to need a big spot for this army to rejoice.

Day 9

Day nine started out bright. I was able to get up and move on my leg, and I ordered a big breakfast, compared with the past days' menus. My ability to mobilize and my outlook seemed even better. The research team said I would begin treatment, and I started preparing for that, but the oncologist decided we needed to postpone treatment until they knew what was going on with my left knee. When the rheumatology and orthopedic physicians came to visit, they said there were no explanations for the swelling and inability to use (or limited mobility); it could be an infection, but no revelation in the cultures had occurred as of yet. White blood cell numbers were still within the normal range, but the bone marrow biopsy did confirm AML. Therefore, the doctor decided to go ahead with treatment … tomorrow. It looked like there would be more of those hurry-up-and-wait days on the books. We continued to draw strength and encouragement from the blog and website; we all laughed and cried together when we read the words from our friends and fellow Christians from near and far.

One of my favorite pastimes has become making the nursing staff and housekeeping staff familiar with some of our South Georgia lingo, which my children refer to as "Claytonisms." When the IV started beeping, I called the nurses' station. When the attendant asked what I needed, I simply said, "This bird dog is barking" or "This bird dog needs you to come see about him." If the IV continued to beep, we pressed some buttons to make it stop. When the nurse came in, I said, "We just fed that bird dog." At first when I called the nurses and talked about the bird dog, there was usually silence on the other end. The nurses and techs had to step down to the room to get clarification. Then it became funny to the ones who had a sense of humor. Some of them, however, needed more than a southern man with a bird dog joke to make them smile. We just shook our heads and laughed.

All the visitors that day were ministers and their wives. They all brought encouraging, uplifting words, saying, "Brother, we need your voice!" in this era of time. I joined in the conversation, agreeing with them that the Word should be proclaimed to this world of lost people and those who have strayed away from the faith they knew they should be living. These fellow soldiers of the cross, those who are serving on the front battlefields, fellow laborers in pastoring, came to proclaim life to a veteran soldier of the cross.

Day 10

We classified day ten as a "bad" day, but we realize it wasn't completely awful but definitely not high on the list of our favorites. From my room, we could hear the medical airlift helicopter land and depart from the rooftop, so we knew there were other people who faced immediate life-threatening situations. We didn't mean to complain and certainly didn't want to portray that this situation was the most horrible thing ever. We simply wanted to chronicle our journey, letting people know that not every day was good, nor was it all bad. Believe us when we say that the comments, text messages, and posts were part of our mental support system. Knowing that our friends dropped by and left notes revealed to us that our family mattered to many people and that our friends were taking us before the throne room of God.

With the uncertainty of medical reports and not knowing whether treatment was being started or what would flare up next, my family decided to follow the directives in Deuteronomy 6, where the children of Israel were told to put the words of the Lord in front of them. Then they could talk about them when they were sitting, when they were eating, when they were walking, and at any other time they were together. My family brought out construction paper and markers, and they wrote out verses of scripture to hang up in room E605 so we would have the promises of God to remind us daily. They posted the following:

> Fear thou not; for I [am] with thee: be not dismayed; for I [am] thy God: I will strengthen thee; yea, I will help thee; yea, I will uphold thee with the right hand of my righteousness. (Isaiah 41:10)

> Heal me, O Lord, and I shall be healed; save me, and I shall be saved: for thou [art] my praise. (Jeremiah 17:14)

> But he [was] wounded for our transgressions, [he was] bruised for our iniquities: the chastisement of our peace [was] upon him; and with his stripes we are healed. (Isaiah 53:5)

> Is any sick among you? let him call for the elders of the church; and let them pray over him, anointing him with oil in the name of the Lord. (James 5:14)

> And the prayer of faith shall save the sick, and the Lord shall raise him up; and if he have committed sins, they shall be forgiven him. (James 5:15)

We believed in the power of prayer, and with faith, we believed nothing would be impossible. By having these scriptures continually in front of us, we focused on the promises from God's Word instead of the doom and gloom on medical reports. Every time my eyes opened, I saw these scriptures in front of my bed, down the walls, and in every empty space. Written on the white board was Ezekiel 16:6. As they changed shifts, the nurses and techs wouldn't erase those words because they knew they were important to us. As I looked around the room, I could see the following:

And when he had called unto [him] his twelve disciples, he gave them power [against] unclean spirits, to cast them out, and to heal all manner of sickness and all manner of disease. (Matthew 10:1)

And all things, whatsoever ye shall ask in prayer, believing, ye shall receive. (Hebrews 11:6)

But without faith [it is] impossible to please [him]: for he that cometh to God must believe that he is, and [that] he is a rewarder of them that diligently seek him. (Matthew 21:22)

Now faith is the substance of things hoped for, the evidence of things not seen. (Hebrews 11:1)

For with God nothing shall be impossible. (Luke 1:37)

That your faith should not stand in the wisdom of men, but in the power of God. (1 Corinthians 2:5)

For we walk by faith, not by sight. (2 Corinthians 5:7)

If ye abide in me, and my words abide in you, ye shall ask what ye will, and it shall be done unto you. (John 15:7)

Therefore I say unto you, What things soever ye desire, when ye pray, believe that ye receive [them], and ye shall have [them]. (Mark 11:24)

And I say unto you, Ask, and it shall be given you; seek, and ye shall find; knock, and it shall be opened unto you. (Luke 11:9)

> [The righteous] cry, and the Lord heareth, and
> delivereth them out of all their troubles. (Psalm
> 34:17)

> Jesus said unto him, If thou canst believe, all things
> [are] possible to him that believeth. (Mark 9:23)

> Be strong and of a good courage, fear not, nor be
> afraid of them: for the Lord thy God, he [it is] that
> doth go with thee; he will not fail thee, nor forsake
> thee. (Deuteronomy 31:6)

They posted a proclamation related to Jeremiah 33:3—"Call unto me, and I will answer thee, and shew thee great and mighty things"—above my bed because they knew it would be an anchor for me in the dark days when it seemed like I was in a fight for my life. That scripture had been a driving force when I pastored at Liberty Faith. We had a banner in our church that said, "Expect great and mighty things from the Lord!" We were definitely expecting the Lord to move in great and mighty ways in E605! It was amazing to watch different hospital workers come into my room, because they always looked around and said they felt comfort, hope, or peace when they entered.

Even though we declared the Word of the Lord, we still had a battle to endure. I spent this day hurting and waiting, waiting and hurting. I was supposed to start the chemo on this day, so I got up early and wanted to take a shower to be ready for whatever challenges were ahead. Due to medications and shift changes, my shower had to wait for almost three hours. Add to that excruciating knee pain worse than previous days. Rheumatology visited me with no new information except that no infection was found, but the chemo was delayed—yet again. Instead, new orders were given, and I waited on more tests: CT scans to determine whether there were sinus infections due to a cough I had developed (which could be dangerous with my nonexistent immunity) and an MRI of my left knee.

My least favorite medical testing machine of any available was the MRI machine. Claustrophobia prevents me from liking an MRI *at all*. So far, there were no infections in the knee, no gout, no injuries; and the doctors were working together to determine what would cause such severe pain and limited mobility. After hurrying to wait all day for these tests, I was finally able to rest, but still on the horizon was the unknown world of chemo treatment. Someone called today, and I told him or her that it was like getting ready for a wedding and waiting at the altar for a girl who didn't show up. (My children said this was another Claytonism.)

The waiting and wondering work out for the good sometimes, and sometimes they don't end so well. If I determined that I didn't really need this treatment now, or if it was going to be bad for my knee and leg, then I wanted it delayed. However, there had to be a reason why the treatment kept being postponed. *Why are we having to spend so much time up here just waiting, Lord?* I wondered. After pondering for a bit, I knew it was all for His glory. *After all, this is all about Him, not about us.* We would take the waiting over worse news any day. This situation made us think of a statement we have all heard so many times: stand still and let God move. If it took standing still, sitting still, or resting still, we had that covered. As a matter of fact, we believed we would *take a front row seat and watch God move.*

Day 11

I felt much better on day eleven, and I believe this was due to the prayers of the people. Everyone gathered in our hospital room had kind of joked about the fact that these days were like a roller—coaster ride, with definite highs and lows, but this was just the beginning of this leg of the trip. So far it had promised to be the ride of our lives.

We were becoming acquainted with various members of the hospital staff, and I couldn't help but make a few jokes to make the days go by with more ease. After all, Proverbs 17:22 tells us, "A merry heart doeth good like a medicine: but a broken spirit drieth the bones." I told my family, "You've got to watch 'em around here like a chicken watches a hawk. You never know when they might be coming for blood, fluid, a test, or information." So they watched the door warily like a hawk, never knowing who was coming in for what.

Late the night before, the nurses had come in and explained that the lab reports indicated that I may need blood products transfused. This information was a definite blow to us this early in the game. We thought that would come later. The children started getting text messages going back and forth—along with phone calls and tears over information about what "could be"—to each of the family members and their spouses. Meanwhile, we let worry ride along this roller coaster for a few minutes. Then together, we did what we knew would give us the comfort we needed: we prayed. We encouraged one another with messages that God was in control and that He could move mountains.

Not many minutes later, I was able to be up, ready to shower, eat breakfast, and face the day ahead. After all, chemo was scheduled for today. Miraculously, lab reports showed that *no blood products were needed*. Praise the Lord! Also, my left knee and leg, which had been causing problems, were feeling so much better. CT scans and the MRI showed no real cause for the left leg pain. Rheumatology and orthopedics decided it could be arthritis—still no infection and no evidence of injury. And they brought word that chemo would be delayed … again. It was very difficult to fathom why the treatment had been delayed so many times. One thing we knew: God had a plan. It was up to us to be submissive and just fight the fight against doubt, fear, and uncertainty. The ride would continue.

As we had realized, this roller-coaster ride had already been full of ups and downs, but *thank God* we didn't have to ride it alone.

It was evident with every turn that we weren't riding alone; we had the Lord, and we had all of our friends, who were checking in with us daily to let us know we weren't alone. We drew so much strength from scripture, especially Isaiah 43:1–2. "But now thus saith the Lord that created thee, O Jacob, and he that formed thee, O Israel, Fear not: for I have redeemed thee, I have called thee by thy name; *thou art mine*. When thou passest through the waters, I will be with thee; and through the rivers, they shall not overflow thee: when thou walkest through the fire, thou shalt not be burned; neither shall the flame kindle upon thee" (emphasis added).

CHAPTER 4

CHEMOTHERAPY, PART 1 (DAYS 12–20)

Day 12

"This is the day," I muttered to myself, hoping I would be cured of the ailment by God's mercy since this was the day we were supposed to start the chemo. The hurry-up-and-wait day started with a bang. I woke up early, showered, shaved, and ate a remarkable breakfast. There were many uncertainties in my mind as I awaited the dreaded chemo. The only thing I knew without any doubt was that God would be with me. We had the typical rounds of nurses, doctors, and techs strolling the hospital corridors. And all these officials wanted to ensure that our questions were answered. With so many concerns, we didn't even know where to begin asking questions.

In all honesty, I was just trusting in the Lord to guide me throughout this special day. Isaiah 12:2 says, "Behold, God is my salvation; I will trust, and not be afraid: for the Lord Jehovah is my strength and my song; he also is become my salvation." And without a doubt, the Lord was at my side every step of the way. When the reports started coming in, we had another day of decent bloodwork. Praise the Lord! I was scheduled to take the first chemo pill at approximately twelve thirty. Everyone kept comforting me, saying that each person reacted differently and that ultimately God would *always* be in control.

As soon as the clock hit the twelve-thirty mark, the EKGs were set up ... the blood work was completed ... and within minutes, the chemo started. The time was finally upon me. I could eat only two hours after taking the first dose. We bowed our heads and prayed humbly, asking God to help me in this moment. I also enjoyed the arrival of numerous visitors, who came to express their concerns, prayers, and encouragement. Some came from as far away as Brunswick. And truth be told, I was pretty amazed by the sacrifices friends made just to show their support for my family and me.

At about six, Sherry asked how I was feeling, and I responded with a Claytonism. "Somewhere between perky and forty." For a person in my position, age sixty-four, these two days were surprisingly good. Moreover, we received several text messages and posts on our blog that said, "Praying continually." This explained what was actually happening; God was hearing the prayers of His people and helping me through the process.

In Acts 12, we find the story of Peter being bound in the inner prison with four quaternions of soldiers to keep him imprisoned, but *the church prayed without ceasing unto God for him.* Peter was bound with chains, sleeping between guards, and had keepers at the door of the prison, yet the way was made. Deliverance came. My children made a plea for the saints of God, fellow soldiers, and warriors of Christ to keep lifting us up, keep standing in the gap, keep approaching the throne, and keep believing God for this miracle, because He was working.

Day 13

The next day was the second day of chemo treatment, and it was a little different from yesterday. The usual activities were routine, and I felt great. At the same time, weekends were turning out to be the most convenient times for visitors, and they flooded the sixth floor. These visitors hailed from far and wide, bringing gifts, donations, prayers, smiles, and encouraging words. Some visitors brought the gift of song, ministering it so other patients wanted to know where that singing was coming from. They murmured to each other, "Is it on some media station?"

"No," the nurses replied. "It's that room over there," referring to my room, E605. While others fought battles with spears and swords, we determined to fight with a tried and true method: praise. Like the children of Israel, there are times when God's people don't have to fight battles utilizing physical weapons. Rather, these people come in the name of the Lord, offering praise to our great God. We proclaimed, "Sickness, depression, oppression, despair, you have no place here. We are singing the praises of our heavenly King!"

My children related to me an amazing story of what happened today when they arrived at the hospital, wearing our uniquely designed T-shirts displaying the slogan "God Said, Live!" My daughter had a vinyl creation business, offering custom shirts and personalized items. When my family exited their vehicles in the parking garage, a man was keenly watching them while leaning against a pole. He asked my family whether they were part of some church group. My family explained that they were wearing the shirts in my support since I had just recently been diagnosed with leukemia.

The man was astonished since his father-in-law was sick, and to encourage his family, one of his family members had sent Ezekiel 16:6 to him in the form of a text. You see, this man's pastor, who was in Honduras on a mission trip, had sent him a scripture by text to minister to the family in this grave period of illness. And this verse was exactly the same, Ezekiel 16:6! You can imagine his bewilderment when they all showed up in the parking area with that same scripture printed on shirts because there was a total of twelve of my family members wearing these shirts. They testified to him about the power in the Word and the Lord's goodness to confirm His Word. You never know to whom you are witnessing when you are just going about your daily activities.

Sometime after the twelve-thirty chemo administration, everything seemed rather fine and under control. The nurses told me they would bring Maalox, if needed, in light of the different aftertastes and acid reflux from the treatment. When the peppermint-flavored medicine arrived, I told them just like my daddy used to say, "Sister Maalox has been a good ole gal all these years!" And, like always, the bird dog (IV machine) was hollering, and I still requested the nurses to come see it. One nurse on that day informed me, "That bird dog is going to be your best friend." People normally refer to a dog as a man's best friend. Right now, this bird dog was definitely a consistent companion. I wondered whether I should give it a name since it was becoming a part of the family.

At about four, I started feeling weak and instantly felt nauseous. Prayer requests were sent out almost immediately on the Remind app and through phone messages. And immediately we started witnessing results of the prayer. One of my conscientious nurses noticed my discomfort and tried to find ways to make me more comfortable.

Then, after a little while, she returned to share the most recent blood work's astonishingly positive results. With tears of joy, she shared the remarkable results with the family. As we discussed the news, we instantly thought of Ezekiel 16:6. "And when I passed by thee, and saw thee polluted in thine own blood, I said unto thee when thou wast in thy blood, Live; yea, I said unto thee when thou wast in thy blood, Live."

The blood work clearly showed that our case had been taken before the throne of God once again. It made me recall one of my favorite songs, "Calvary Still Touches Me."

All things considered, I can honestly say that I felt the touch of Calvary on that day. I wasn't running circles around the hospital, but I had this hope, and of this we are sure: "We are troubled on every side, yet not distressed; we are perplexed, but not in despair; Persecuted, but not forsaken; cast down, but not destroyed" (2 Corinthians 4:8–9). These verses couldn't possibly depict our feelings any better. Bad news may seem to pop up from out of nowhere in a desperate attempt to flood our hearts with fear and worry at every bump in the road, although I was glad that neither me nor my family was in despair. Our trust remains in God, who has never done us anything but good.

Day 14

This day, which was a Sunday, marked the end of two weeks in the hospital. Frankly, my stay actually felt like two months. Since I still had to spend several weeks, I became somewhat quieter and reflective. My family all sympathized with me, understanding how much I loved home and church services. This was the third weekend I hadn't been able to be in church. In the past, the longest I could remember not being in church was maybe ten days.

It seemed as if we were about to shatter that record. However, not being present "in a church building" had certainly not prevented us from "having church." We continued to feel His presence on the sixth floor every day, confirming that a mighty work was being done. For we knew that Matthew recorded in letters of red, "Where two or three are gathered together in my name, there am I in the midst of them" (Matthew 18:20). We have no doubt that the Almighty was there!

This was, in effect, the third day of chemotherapy. I did undergo some uncomfortable symptoms but nothing severe. Nausea attempted to invade the room throughout the day. Because this was the thing I dreaded the most, it may be why I noticed it more than anything else. To keep things on the lighter side with everyone, when I felt the onset of nausea, I informed the nurse, "I feel Goosey," another well-known Claytonism. Moreover, my taste buds had seemed to jump ship, although I still pushed myself to eat, knowing I needed the nourishment for the coming days. My skin started feeling strange, almost as if it were drying up and on the verge of being peeled off. It was an unusual feeling, but I considered it to be one more thing I had to deal with.

In the afternoon, I was moved to a different room. One of the techs who claimed to oversee the room assignments informed me that he was holding a special room for me down the hall and around the corner. Because the room was on the other side of the wing, the view had dramatically improved. The room overlooked a large green soccer field and Emory University with Atlanta skyscrapers in the background.

It also felt like it was a little bit bigger than my other room; this fact was great considering all the family members who came to visit. After entering the room, I was again amazed by the favor God had bestowed on me in the form of physicians, nurses, and staff at the hospital. My children attributed my blessings to the many times I showed appreciation for all the medical staff's efforts and my attempt at humor by speaking in parables. One of the wonderful nurses brought me some TED hose or stockings (thromboembolism deterrent). Those are really tight, white stockings patients are asked to wear to prevent blood clots. After noticing the tights, I immediately told her, "That looks like my granny's stockings! I'm not sure that I want to wear those." My son Terry took them from the nurse as the entire family laughed and girded me up.

Before long, it was time to read the comments on my blog and get our daily dose of encouragement. The kind remarks had always offered us such strength, since we knew we weren't alone in our fight. The scriptures and testimonies were like an oasis in a parching desert. I knew the next day would bring even more trying battles because the medical staff had instructed me that IV induction chemotherapy would commence the following morning. It would be a regular twelve-hour infusion for at least a week. Once again, we would face the unknown, and we were clinging to Hebrews 13:6. "So that we may boldly say, The Lord is my helper, and I will not fear what man shall do unto me."

Day 15

This day awakened us even before the sun. I knew there would be a big day ahead. At about six a.m., I felt that the Lord impressed some words on my heart, which I wanted to share personally with the people on the blog rather than through my children. They decided to record me speaking and upload the video to a YouTube channel. They also asked everyone to pray throughout the day as the induction chemo was about to begin.

That day was undoubtedly the real deal. Not to belittle any days before, but we were aware that this day could be somewhere between great and/or disastrous. One type of chemo was ingested in fifteen minutes, but the other was to be infused all day for over twenty-four hours. We were originally told that it would last no more than twelve hours. However, later down the line, we found out it had to be done for the full twenty-four hours.

For one entire week, I did twenty-four hours of chemo every single day! Despite this confusion, we felt God had answered our prayers since this treatment was more than tolerable for now. Because of this, we continued praising Him throughout the day. With so many uncertainties, we did all we knew to do—depend on the One who knows all things. He was the One to rely on. Like Job, we believed that "he knoweth the way that I take: when he hath tried me, I shall come forth as gold" (Job 23:10).

I felt surprisingly good. I couldn't let anyone forget my bird dog IV pole, and it stayed with me throughout. I still didn't assign a name to it. Around lunchtime (nearly two thirty), I told Terry my taste buds were reacting better. The two buds that were left had been dancing around, trying to avoid each other. That was my way of saying that the food tasted better. One of my food items was a sweet potato, and it tasted far better than it looked. I informed Terry that they had put the hammer down on this sweet potato. It was so funny to see the look on the nurses' faces as they tried to decipher my Clayton code.

Nearly every hour or so, we took a portion of time to read the blog comments, since they were a great distraction from the humming of the machines and the dripping of the IV medication. Often we were laughing, sometimes crying, but we were gaining strength with each passing moment. As I got a double dose of chemotherapy on day fifteen, I felt like giving a double dose of words for the blog. I had already made a video. Then I decided to send a personal message for the blog, which Terry specifically transcribed for me. This personal message read as follows:

> I just wanted to say, "Praise the Lord" for great friends, great family, and a remarkable church family! We started today with many concerns about the new chemotherapy medications. How would we react to them? Praise the Lord, following the therapy, we only had minor problems. Nothing a great God Jehovah couldn't fix! Now we believe in the God of Abraham, Isaac, and Jacob!

> There is still no fear of leaving this world that I have called home for the last sixty-four years. My joy becomes greater whenever I reflect on these things. Isaiah 40:29 says, "He giveth power to the faint; and to them that have no might he increaseth strength." This is where I am right now. Sinner, this time will come in your life when you are weak and will not have life in you. By faith in Jesus Christ,

you can say, "He hath given me the power instead of weakness" and "given strength when I had no might."

Tomorrow will be Tuesday, another round of chemotherapy, and more things to take into consideration. But let me tell you that my peace has never been greater as we fight on for our cause to come before our Father's throne. Please keep the faith with my family and myself. Remember Ezekiel 16:6.

It is so vital for us to keep the faith, no matter what battle we are facing. Believe, no matter what the odds have become. Strive, no matter how difficult the situation may be. And do not ever back up on what is right, for He will give you power and strength if you fear not. This conviction was so embedded in me that I wanted to run through a troop and leap over a wall.

Who but God can do such things as these?

Day 16

This was the second day of intensive IV chemotherapy, and it proved far better than the first. Even though I was weak, I didn't have any severe challenges. God kept nausea, vomiting, headaches, GI symptoms, and so forth all at bay. It was almost as if there was a wall built out of prayers surrounding me. I felt like I was covered completely with the prayers of the saints. This was a shield far stronger than tempered steel or Kevlar. It could withstand all the fiery darts of the adversary. So many prayers had been sent up on my behalf, so there was much intercession for my healing, and the enemy didn't have a place to camp and attack. With the help garnered through prayer, meditation, fasting, obedience, visits, calls, and messages, we persistently asked God for better days to continue. I can honestly say I couldn't have made it through these days so easily without the prayers and support of our friends and family.

The previous night, a nurse shared that the nursing staff rarely saw someone with family and friends' support, which they constantly noticed in my room. When the doctor came by today (only two visitors allowed at the time), she smiled and said, "Your room is always full of visitors and family."

She looked around the room, seeing all the scriptures taped to the walls on red construction paper, and recognized this room was full not only of people but also of God's Word. Romans 10:17 states, "So then faith cometh by hearing, and hearing by the word of God." So we had the words of God right where they could be read and reread, because through our hearing, believing, it results in faith. His Word is the key!

One nurse informed us of a young adult patient, who had no support whatsoever. Only a few days into his treatment, he was found crying in his room. Deeply scarred from the loneliness, desolate from the solitude, and unable to bear the load of his illness alone, he was desperately asking for his mother. He was looking for someone to show compassion, maybe pray, or just be present with him in his difficult journey. Bearing this in mind, I was so glad for our family—not only the Morgans but also all our brothers and sisters in Christ.

We obtained the evening blood test results, and it brought even more good news to the family. According to the reports, we were inching farther away from getting transfusions. A typical transfusion is composed of packed red blood cells and platelets. We knew that ten to fourteen days after starting the IV chemotherapy, it was a pretty standard procedure. However, we also knew without a doubt that God was keeping everything on His balance sheet. The nurse entered my room again on that day and exclaimed astonishingly, "His levels are continuously getting better—this is so unusual."

We knew the reason, and we were telling it to everyone (whether he or she was interested or not). My friend, there is power, power, wonder-working power in the blood of the Lamb. He met us at every turn, helped us to maneuver over every obstacle, and gave us strength like never before.

With this positive note, another day was completed. The battle was still being fought. However, the finish line had become one day closer. And in all honesty, the preacher in me desperately needed a pulpit. In fact, my children informed me that, on that very day, I said to a nurse that we would pray for her "Pentecostal style." In any case, one thing was for sure; as soon as I was going to get discharged from Emory University Hospital, my congregation required a picnic lunch because I would be preaching longer than they were accustomed.

Day 17

Day three of induction chemotherapy was, in effect, day seventeen in my grueling struggle against AML. The day started off strangely. My son Mark was staying on a cot in the room with me. My children had purchased it so family members could take turns staying so I wouldn't be alone. As soon as Mark woke up, he got up and headed straight toward the shower. During that time, the nurse call button turned on out of nowhere, with the nurse on the other end asking, "Can I help you?" I responded by telling her that I didn't need anything. Then, after a few minutes, the nurse call button went off again and again. I kept informing the hospital staff that I didn't need anything. Before long, a nurse came down to the room because, according to him, I was calling them.

Upon closer examination, the nurse realized that Mark had put his duffel bag on the pull cord in the bathroom. This had triggered the nurse call light, which had convinced the nurses' station that I needed assistance. After solving the mystery, we all had a good laugh, and we were glad that we had something that had lightened the mood. When Mark apologized to the nursing staff, I told him I was thinking about something crazy. When he asked what craziness I had in mind, I told him, "Ice cream and dill pickles!"

Mark dutifully remarked, "If you will eat that, I can get them right now. It isn't far from the hospital. It will take me no time."

I jokingly replied, "No way!" We had a few laughs, although they were rather short lived since this was about the time when many questions began coming.

After a while, we received another blood work report. It indicated that my blood sugar was extremely high, my fever was above normal levels, and I was experiencing some tightness in my chest. At the same time, my nausea had resurfaced, and it was making its presence known. The tightness in my chest required immediate action to find its root cause. Before long, I had a nurse sticking leads to my chest for a stat EKG. From that point on, I began wondering exactly how that day would play out.

There was no doubt that the walls of prayer had protected us every day at the hospital, and on this particular day we needed them more than anything else. To help us spiritually in these troubling moments, Mark's wife sent us these words from her devotion: Psalm 18:1–2 says, "I will love thee, O Lord, my strength. The Lord is my rock, and my fortress, and my deliverer; my God, my strength, in whom I will trust; my buckler, and the horn of my salvation, and my high tower." In all honesty, we found this verse extremely relevant and true to our situation. Even when it appeared that everything was turning from us, we found God delivering on His promise once again. Thankfully, the EKG came back normal, my fever plummeted, and I began eating yogurt and Jell-O.

I was aware that the "sky juice" (my code name for IV chemotherapy) would bring days like that. The most important thing was that we had Someone we could call on in the midnight hour. We had Someone we could depend on, no matter what was brewing inside and around us. Most of all, we had Someone who would answer the "call light," whether we called on Him or someone else called.

In our battle, we found God coming to our rescue time and time again. So many people pushed the call button of heaven on our behalf, and we are indebted to them from the bottoms of our hearts. We were glad He was an on-time God. He will hold our hand and deliver us from all evil at every turn.

As the uncertain day was near its end, my phone buzzed with a text from a preacher friend who had stayed in close contact with me. He told me to recite Psalms 119:50. "This is my comfort in my affliction: for thy word hath quickened me." What words to lean on! With fever raging, anxiety increasing, and no appetite, we knew the Word of God would quicken us and prove to be our rock in this midnight hour. We kept hoping the next day would be a better day.

Day 18

Day 18 brought us more new experiences. There was so much going on all the time. We needed this test, we required that result, we needed vital signs, we needed lab reports, we needed weight, we needed food orders, and we needed to tell the doctor. I teasingly told my family, "You get too much candy for a dime around here!"

Along with the normal stuff, we struggled to comprehend new procedures and medicines and how each impacted the body. We tried to sift through what was expected and unexpected and tried our best not to jump on and off the roller coaster of fear and worry.

The moment I woke up on day eighteen, a nurse tech entered the room, and I casually asked her, "Do you believe the Word of the Lord, sis?"

An apparent glow came over her face as she responded, "Yes, sir, I do." This was just one instance while at Emory when I asked someone a question regarding the Lord. I considered this to be an everyday part of conversation. What's more, I believe we must mention the Lord and His goodness as much as we can, which I believe is part of the Great Commission. Some of these nurses and techs came to understand what made me a little different from other patients. One person even told his coworkers that if he disappeared from off the floor working, he would be in our room, "getting his witness on."

With one of the nurses, I discussed Sarah and the promises that seemed far away. However, we must understand that God's timetable doesn't always have to comply with our wishes. Sarah doubted God and had trouble believing God would fulfill His promises, so she just developed her own solution to her situation. Countless times, we find it challenging to wait for God to act in our situation. The wait appears to be the hardest task we have ever faced. Is it that we become dissatisfied with God's solution because we find it unjust according to our understanding?

To better understand this scenario, let's examine what God instructed Abraham in Genesis 18:14. "Is anything too hard for the Lord?" If you are going through a battle that seems too hard to win or facing a mountain too hard to climb, you must ask yourself, Is there anything too difficult for our God?

Even in Atlanta, Georgia, surrounded by the best health care money can buy, human nature allowed us to ask questions like, "Why am I suffering?" or "Why does my family have to suffer?" Is it because there is a nurse or doctor somewhere who must see a miracle? Is there a backslider somewhere who needs to realize this one particular voice, which has always called out his or her name in prayer, can be silenced for a time? Personally, I have always liked the song that says, "Fix it like you want it, Lord; it's alright with me!" It has always been my desire for the Lord to use me for the upbuilding His kingdom. I say let it be done according to Your will.

We know that for such a time as this we are where God wants us to be. So, Lord, let our words, thoughts, actions, and reactions line up according to what would be pleasing to You. Is the Lord using my life to unfold an extraordinary plan? God can prove He isn't limited to what normally happens. We have already seen the hand of God move in areas outside the normality of science.

Blood levels improved just as if a pint of blood had been given. However, no blood products were hanging by the bed or being administered by the nursing team. Rather, we believe the blood came from another Source, a source not limited by science. Day by day, we watched God's plan unfold. We were beginning to see firsthand the unlimited options that are elements of the package. Is anything too hard for the Lord?

Day 19

Much like the previous day, this one had its fair share of new experiences. The bird dog had so many hookups that the hospital staff had to introduce new hardware/software to keep it running smoothly. The bird dog required high maintenance, requiring almost constant attention. If you feel that beagles and hound dogs on the farm cause a lot of racket, just get hooked up to one of these little doggies, which have more than six lines of various fluids going at scheduled times. Whenever one fluid runs out, "The bird dog starts barking."

The nurses' desk was now aware that it was probably the bird dog whenever our room's buzzer made a noise, so they automatically sent someone to check it out. This morning, when Becky's phone alarm turned on, I thought it was the bird dog and immediately rang the nurses' station. Brenda was the one who informed me that, at that time, it wasn't the bird dog but Becky's phone alarm. It was so early; we all desperately wanted the noise to stop because we had been awake on and off ever since four a.m. The nurses were trying to obtain accurate blood levels to determine whether I required a blood transfusion.

Having never gone through these circumstances before, it seemed to be a terrifying experience for my family and me. The nurse kept reassuring us that once I received the blood, I would, in fact, feel better. It surprises me how our minds can change about something and how we can look at things with a different perspective when circumstances force us to do so. I wanted to wait until the last possible moment before needing blood products, and I reached this point early on that morning.

I had previously been a blood donor, but I had never been a recipient of blood. At this point, we became very appreciative of everyone who had ever given blood, for every organization that had blood drives, and for the individuals who organized and conducted these drives. I had felt so poorly the previous day, and we had to act based on the current blood levels. I was left with no appetite to speak of and no energy to do anything but sleep. The nurse kept informing us that the blood had been ordered, but we weren't sure how that would work.

Nevertheless, the difference I felt after receiving the blood was truly amazing. Initially, I had a fever, and blood cultures were still being examined to find the fever's cause. Lab reports were consulted, and the white blood count numbers were exactly what they expected. This part of the report received several cheers and clapping from the nurses.

By midmorning, the fever went down, and they were finally able to order and prepare for the transfusion. This was another routine: hurry up, get it scheduled, and then ... another wait-for-it-to-arrive moment. Throughout much of the afternoon, with the blood going into my body, my color improved, according to my family, and I felt stronger. The nurses were glad to be able to give me the transfusion because they knew it would make me feel better. Nausea became a constant companion, though, along with the lack of appetite for any real food. Despite this, I cherished the blog comments and guest book entries that day as soon as my family shared them.

At the same time, some family and friends visited and brightened up our entire day. Reflecting on the past two days, I remember they were remarkable battles, struggles I had never experienced before. Day nineteen was also Brenda's birthday, and we wanted to celebrate it with some form of festivities. Becky found birthday cake at one of the hospital's storefronts, so we had somewhat of a mini celebration with a couple of visitors who had stopped by.

The events of the day made me think about blood and what it meant to us. When the nurse brought in the first unit of blood, I expressed to her that life is definitely in the blood, speaking from both a literal and spiritual sense. On a physical level, we must have blood to live. For our organs to function properly and for us to even breathe deeply and experience the very basis of life, we require blood—blood that is free from any harmful disease and toxins. From a spiritual standpoint, we also require blood, which cleanses us from sin.

All this talk about the blood brought to my mind numerous scriptures about blood and its significance to us Christians. As the physical blood offers us a visual reminder of the significance of the blood flowing in our natural bodies, I sat up and searched for the scriptures that talked about blood. In all my sixty-four years, I never required the physical blood of another human being, yet it became necessary for life on day nineteen.

Friend, you may be thinking that you have never needed the blood of anyone else until this point in your life as well. The children of Israel received instructions from Moses on how to escape destruction in Egypt, and we use the same application today to represent our salvation experience. Exodus 12:13 reads, "And the *blood* shall be to you for a token upon the houses where ye are: and when I see the *blood*, I will pass over you, and the plague shall not be upon you to destroy you, when I smite the land of Egypt" (emphasis added).

I wonder if you have the blood applied to your heart for the life of Jesus to flow through you. John 6:53 says, "Then Jesus said unto them, Verily, verily, I say unto you, Except ye eat the flesh of the Son of man, and drink his *blood*, ye have no life in you" (emphasis added). And also 1 John 1:7: "But if we walk in the light, as he is in the light, we have fellowship one with another, and the *blood* of Jesus Christ his Son cleanseth us from all sin" (emphasis added). For us to have life, we *must* have blood, both physically and spiritually. So I ask you, do you have the blood applied to your life?

Day 20

At around 4:30 a.m. on Saturday, March 1, I woke up to shower, shave, and get ready to meet my grandchildren. They normally stayed in the waiting room, where they could all be together. While together, they enjoyed sitting, laughing, talking, and sometimes writing songs or making up some kind of program designed to cheer me up. I felt wonderful—no pain to speak of, no fever, and limited nausea.

Following breakfast, visitors began arriving from home. We then made our way to the designated waiting area, dragging that bird dog (IV pole) with us. In the waiting room, other visitors joined us as well, and things progressed quite nicely, just chatting and laughing. At some point, we discussed the advantages of having the PICC line, and I described it as the "A-artery." I am aware that this isn't an accurate medical term. However, it was of tremendous help, considering all the blood, medicines, and treatments that could be administered through it.

We visited with our grandchildren for a while. They always sang to me and usually wrote special verses to songs that declared the healing power of God. They even joyfully told me they were ready for me to return to the farm so I could make some homemade ice cream. Quite frankly, I was really happy they had come to see me. Here is another YouTube link of one of their special songs: https://www.youtube.com/watch?v=vSgcaZ7krB8&t=18s.

It was difficult for them to stay contained in the waiting area while their parents were visiting me on the other wing. Now add in the fact that they were seeing me in this scary mask and hospital gown. Moreover, my grandchildren weren't allowed to touch me because I couldn't get close to germs. That was the only way the medical team even allowed me to visit with them. As a result, we were left with no choice but to embrace gigantic air hugs. I told them I loved them very much and wanted them to continue living for the Lord, no matter the cost.

When it was time for the chemo treatment, we went back to the room, and still more visitors came, ambassadors from the Lord, bringing encouraging words to all of us. At around 4 p.m., soon after the last group of visitors' departures, the day started, heading in a seemingly different direction. It was time to ride that roller coaster of uncertainty again. I guess the enemy of my soul didn't want me to experience any joy or happiness for a substantial period.

From this point on, the words here contain details I got from my children. There were times when my fever was so high and my pain and nausea so great that I didn't have lucid thoughts. It was impossible for me to pray, much less participate in conversations about what was happening.

My fever increased instantaneously, nausea crept in, and pain started flaring up in my abdomen. How could this happen so quickly? Before we could get turned around, my fever was over 104. My family sent out prayer requests, and even part of the medical staff joined us in prayer as my family requested God to cool the fever. Within a few minutes, the fever began receding. My children thought we could breathe easier, and we did for a short period. Then I started coughing and suffered from a shortness of breath that wasn't previously present. This was a new thing to be concerned about. More prayer requests were sent out. We knew God had heard our prayers, and we were trusting in Him to calm the entire situation.

Throughout this entire ordeal, we had reached a definite conclusion. In this large sea of people in the metropolitan city, in this vast conglomeration of concrete and asphalt, in this jumble of highways and junctions, in this maze of hallways and walls, God proved again on day twenty that He knew exactly where we were.

He showed us that we were on His mind and that He was working a mighty wonder. Some of His people sent texts and called us, while others posted messages on our blog and other social media sites as "a great cloud of witnesses" (Hebrews 12:1), ensuring us that this journey was possible. Some of His people came to visit us to let us know we had been on their minds and in their hearts. And they had been petitioning heaven for my healing. Some of His people, our brothers and sisters in Christ, joined my family in prayer as we battled against sickness, fever, and pain.

Still others brought us direct messages from the Lord, affirming that He had this situation under control. I can assure you that there is nothing like hearing directly from someone who has been interceding on our behalf, taking our case before the almighty mercy seat of heaven! The night looked dark, but we were holding onto the promise of God. Psalm 18:6 says, "In my distress, I called upon the Lord, and cried unto my God: he heard my voice out of his temple, and my cry came before him, even into his ears."

CHAPTER 5

DAY 21

There is no doubting the fact that the number twenty-one has quickly turned into the most significant number for my family, the Morgans. I believe its importance will prevail for many years to come. Why do I say this? I say this because our twenty-first day at Emory was by far the most memorable event in my existence. On that day, we truly saw the hand of God at work. I was so completely out of touch with all that was going on that the details given here are my firsthand experiences, as relayed to me by my family.

In all honesty, every bit of emotion and faith we could muster was packed into these twenty-four hours. The fever from the day before carried over into day twenty-one, Sunday, with a mighty fury. I made an attempt to wake up at about 4:30 a.m. However, as soon as I got up out of bed, I knew I was too weak to make it back to the bed. After calling for assistance, it frankly seemed that everything was going downhill from there.

In a short while, I received news that my blood pressure was high, and I began trembling viciously while suffering from shortness of breath. My voice shook so much that family members who had stayed with me overnight couldn't understand what I was saying. And unfortunately during this time, the fever didn't subside for a single moment.

Seeing my temperature, the nurse brought in a cooling pad or blanket. However, despite her many attempts, the fever still persisted. Becky called the other siblings who had stayed at local motels or at local holiness churches, which had so graciously opened the doors of their evangelist facilities, and they all arrived around 6 a.m. and huddled in groups around the room and in the waiting room. Throughout the morning, my family prayed and sent out requests with the aid of the Remind app and quick personal text messages. I, on the other hand, was in a state of utter confusion. I couldn't understand what was happening. The nurse told us she had done everything she could to bring down the fever. After saying this, she joined hands with my family around my bedside and prayed with them for the Lord to move.

According to my family, they began to discuss and proclaim the words previously spoken. *Things are not as dark as they seem.* My family was sure God would touch me, but they didn't know exactly how or when. Prayers for my well-being were going up from all over the United States. My children received text messages that this church and that church was praying for our family. They knew it was only a matter of time before something remarkable was going to happen. At the same time, hundreds of participants at a youth conference in Alabama stretched their hands across the aisles just to join hands and pray together for me. A church family member and fellow minister called and felt led to pray with my family on speakerphone, coming against this fever that was making me feel so terrible. Hell was fighting our family, and we were clinging to the promises of God.

After a while, my family stepped out of the room for a few minutes and talked with a nurse, asking her whether she had seen cases similar to mine. They were curious whether our situation was somewhat normal or whether there was information we needed to know. We had never been in this situation before, and never had we faced such a devastating foe. Would this AML, this blood disease, this destroyer indeed win?

The answer from that nurse became seared on their hearts to this day. She affirmed what my family already knew in their hearts. She stated, "You cannot compare your case with the one in this room [pointing next door] or that room [pointing to a different one] or that room [pointing to other rooms around us]. The dynamics in your room are different from these other rooms. You have faith in this room! *The outcome will be different here than in the others!*" Within an hour of that conversation, the dynamics proved true.

My family reported that I stopped shivering and shaking. My temperature started declining tremendously, and I started laughing and joking with other people in the room. As soon as I gained my composure and cracked my first joke, the relief on all my family's faces became evident. Phones were buzzing as text messages came in, asking about me.

My children updated the Remind app and sent out individual texts to people to make everyone aware of my improved condition. Then, in a matter of seconds, the praise reports were being exchanged. As my family spread the good news of my improvement, our friends and extended family members responded with words of praise and adoration to the Lord. They began rejoicing in the good news that God had extended His grace and healing touch to me.

Fortunately, I had many friends who daily, at specific moments, went into their prayer closets and prayed for my good health and speedy recovery. Those friends regularly messaged just to know my specific needs so they could take those needs before the throne of God.

Exodus 15:11 states, "Who is like unto thee, O Lord, among the gods? Who is like thee, glorious in holiness, fearful in praises, doing wonders?" Indeed, who is like the Lord? Just two hours before, we weren't sure what was going to happen. Within one hour, my fever broke, and I began joking and rejoicing with my people. My health had improved so drastically that I got up, took a shower, shaved, got dressed, and visited my grandchildren in the waiting room.

When the nurse asked whether I wanted to wait and take a shower later so I could rest and recover from the turmoil, I replied like Clayton for a second time. "Ain't no need in waiting. Stink is growing!" I think my family was laughing and crying at the same time. We couldn't help but shed tears of joy and offer praise to God for blessing me. Because of this, my family sent out texts, informing everyone of the good news and that God had moved and showered His good graces. In all honesty, the difference was astounding. Down the hall, I went to see nine of my ten grandchildren. Still we proclaim, "Who is like the Lord?"

Let's talk more about day twenty-one. I know someone involved in a battle for twenty-one days, the prophet Daniel. Daniel 10:12–13 reveals, "Then said he unto me, Fear not, Daniel: for from the first day that thou didst set thine heart to understand, and to chasten thyself before thy God, thy words were heard, and I am come for thy words. But the prince of the kingdom of Persia withstood me one and twenty days: but, lo, Michael, one of the chief princes, came to help me." God's answer to Daniel arrived after he prayed for a total of twenty-one days. And there was a battle instigated by the prince of the kingdom of Persia. However, archangel Michael intervened and aided Daniel. Just because the answer or help didn't come quickly, Daniel didn't find a reason to give up and quit praying.

Our battle with this sickness may not have resulted in swift answers, but we didn't give in. We knew our Lord heard us the first day we called. We could say this because Ephesians 6:12 reminds us, "We wrestle not against flesh and blood, but against principalities, against powers, against the rulers of the darkness of this world." And without a doubt, it seemed as if we had wrestled with the fever sickness, which was so determined to bring down my spirit, destroy my mind and body, and devastate the peace and assurance of my family.

But on that day, reinforcements had arrived. The fever, tremors, and weakness were pushed back … on the twenty-first day. Can't you just see God dispatching an angel to take care of the troublesome sickness buffeting one of His servants? God knew where we were as He reaffirmed His presence the day before. All we had to do was ask Him to take care of the situation and trust Him to do it—and He did. So yet again, while receiving His divine touch and surviving another tumultuous day, I find myself posing the question to you all: "Who is like the Lord?"

CHAPTER 6

CHEMOTHERAPY, PART 2 (DAYS 22–26)

Day 22

We spent Monday, March 3, resting and relaxing in the goodness of the Lord, keeping in mind that this wasn't a vacation but resting as much as one possibly can in the hospital. Our nurse was extremely busy between the oral medications that were ordered and the IV medications that were required. The bird dog was always barking about something, finishing up antibiotics, antifungal medication, or some of the blood products. At times, the bird dog acted more like a bulldog— persisting in trying to get someone's attention, which resulted in calls to the nurses' desk.

That particular day reminded me of raising our children on the family farm. During certain hot summer days when we were raising our children after working on whatever latest project was at hand, there was nothing as fun as going for a cool swim in our pond, which was fed by a natural spring. Some of us dove right in over our heads, splashing everyone and everything that was close, while others just kind of played around the shallow parts, glad to be in the coolness. Such was the feeling that reigned after three weeks at Emory, just enjoying the coolness of peace and comfort after the great, hot battle of the previous day.

About 5 a.m., I woke up and started asking for water, then ice water, and drinking several big cups. After the parched feeling I had been experiencing over the past few days, that cool, refreshing water was one of the very things I needed. Fever, shaking, trembling weakness—I had none to speak of. King Solomon described our feelings exactly in 1 Kings 8:23. "And he said, Lord God of Israel, there is no God like thee, in heaven above, or on earth beneath, who keepest covenant and mercy with thy servants that walk before thee with all their heart."

This song, written by our good friend Brother Nathan Johnson, seemed to perfectly parallel the past forty-eight hours for us here at Emory.

> I walked through a desert, so hot and so dry,
> I wondered if I'd ever see water again.
> But God, in His goodness, has brought me to a river.
> And He said, Follow Me and I'll lead you in.
> And I said Thanks be to God, which causes us to triumph—
> Always and in every place!
> On the mountains, in the valleys—
> It doesn't matter to Him,
> For He will be God any way!

He and his wife visited us and sang these words, standing around my hospital bed, the day before I experienced this great "fever desert." Just forty-eight hours ago, it was so hot and dry. Nevertheless, we had the assurance that He would lead us to a river, causing us to triumph, for He would be God anyway.

It is amazing how God makes provisions for us before we even know what lies ahead. Isaiah 41:17–18 records, "When the poor and needy seek water, and there is none, and their tongue faileth for thirst, I the Lord will hear them, I the God of Israel will not forsake them. I will open rivers in high places, and fountains in the midst of the valleys: I will make the wilderness a pool of water, and the dry land springs of water." It seemed that the Lord had opened a river, or pool, or spring for us. We chose to rest in the knowledge that He had a greater plan and purpose for us than we had ever hoped or dreamed of.

As we experienced each day, each blog post, text message, and phone call was like a cool drink of water along our journey, a rest break in the battle we fought against the enemy of sickness and defeat. I listened as people shared testimonies of renewed faith and hope because of the goodness of God they had personally witnessed in our room or from the many posts about our circumstances.

One of the nurses shared with Brenda and me that she knew why we were at Emory. It was for her to see that real faith does exist. She had experienced some form of church hurt in years past and had left her faith, but now her faith had been renewed. She declared that seeing the genuine faith shared by our family had brought her back to a place where she could trust in God again. Our hearts were so touched and moved by this declaration.

It's so important for people to share testimonies of faith, healing, and hope. You never know who may need to know that you have been an overcomer and that it is possible to have victory through the help and grace of God. We just soaked up the refreshing water of ease, not worrying about a fever, nausea, or chemo for at least one day. I did require platelets and two units of blood, but I had no reactions or problems. Even these were nothing to worry about. Thanks be to God! He took care of us each day, proving that He would take care of tomorrow, too. Anybody thirsty? I know where there is water.

Day 23

The last bag of IV chemo was taken down at about 9:22 a.m. on day twenty-three. We reported no major incidents, but we did meet a new member of the doctor team, and he told us that everything was still on track, even though we had to postpone chemo one day because of the fever. I needed two more units of blood, and fever was knocking on our door. (It's amazing to think that "having to get two units of blood" isn't a major incident. Previously, we had thought having to get blood was a major crisis.) Within fifteen minutes of asking people to pray for the fever to be gone, all traces of it disappeared. From that point on, it seemed that it would soon be over in just a few more hours. I slept through most of the day, and we could all rest somewhat easily, knowing this part of the journey was over.

It is almost like your birthday. You wait and wait for it to finally arrive, and yes, you are older; but it is just another day. As far as feelings, the thing that was different was that we had seen for ourselves that it *could* be done; this mountain could be climbed. We know we weren't the first ones to experience this, but now that we have experienced it, we want to add our voices to the ones who say, "You can overcome!"

From the time I woke up, I apparently gave plenty of Claytonisms for the family and the nurses to laugh about. I told the nurse that not everyone could handle that "sky juice" (liquid chemo) as she was checking the IV; that bird dog needed lots of attention today. I had been wearing an oxygen tube since Sunday morning, and I labeled it my "hair clasp," because it went around my ears and bothered them.

When they tried to read me some of the messages from various social media posts, I told Brenda we needed to get something so we could log into the *Home Page Journal* (blog). We weren't up to date on the forms of modern technology, but I could see how much it was helping our souls stay encouraged and how it was keeping people updated with our latest developments.

I decided day twenty-three was a good day to describe some of my boyhood-neighborhood growing-up stories to some of the nurses and techs. And I am sure they will never forget some of the things they had heard from this South Georgia boy. I got into some interesting scrapes when I was a young fellow hanging out with all my buddies.

A nursing staff member, who worked on our side of the hall several of the days we had been at Emory, reported back for duty on this particular day. Since we had not seen her, I asked her where she had been, and she told me she had peeked in earlier, looking for something. I asked, "What were you looking for—a corpse?"

"Not in here!" she replied. "Didn't he say to them bones, 'Live'? I ain't gonna find no corpse in here! No, sir, they gone live!"

We couldn't agree more! I knew she was referring to the dry bones, but it once again reminded me of Ezekiel 16:6. "And when I passed by thee, and saw thee polluted in thine own blood, I said unto thee when thou wast in thy blood, Live; yea, I said unto thee when thou wast in thy blood, Live." We are still proclaiming the promise given in the beginning—"Live!" I shared a saying with my family that goes something like this: You cannot lose with the plan we use. The only outcome for a Christian is on the winning side. You will always come out a winner if you put your trust in the Lord. Some people want to put their hopes in a little of this and a little of that, but we must completely surrender to the Lord. You cannot lose with the plan we use.

Day 24

Fever and weakness threatened our morning from the onset of day twenty-four, but we were able to get it under control. My room was like a revolving door, with nurses, doctors, physicians' assistants, research coordinators, and other technicians having to wait their turn in the hall to get their opportunity to complete whatever procedure was ordered next. I had CT Scans, X-rays, breathing treatment, a new PICC line "installed," more than one EKG, and blood labs drawn. I was very drowsy all day, and I thought it was from all the medications. Since I had no immune system, I had to take antibiotics, antifungal, and other medications to keep from getting infections. I asked for two different foods: fried chicken and an ice cream cone. I hadn't been eating much, and my children were glad to find them for me. I didn't eat much of either one, but it was good to have something I liked. We were still trucking right along with the oral chemo drug, and we had several days of that left. I remember being extremely glad to be done with the IV chemo.

A new nurse came in to check the barking bird dog, and while waiting to be unhooked, I told her I wanted to go for a swim. She looked around, with a questioning look on her face, so my children had to interpret for her that I wanted to take a shower. Since I still had medications to finish, I had to postpone the shower. Another nurse asked me what I was doing because I was snoring while she was taking care of the bird dog. I told her I was playing a little game. When she asked what kind of game, I told her it was one where you read the backs of your eyelids. I did quite a bit of that at Emory.

We had been told in this process that they must tear down everything, kill the bad cells, and build everything up again. We were glad to be on this side of the tearing down. Even though I was still taking the chemo pill, the doctors, nurses, and techs did what they could to build me back up physically. Through this entire process, both have been present: the tearing down and the building up.

When my family first found out there was something terribly wrong with me physically, faith immediately rose up, and we said, "God can handle this," while at the same time, the destroyer or doubter was there to add his thoughts. The enemy of our souls wanted to tear our faith down, but we instilled in our children from the time they were young that God said, "But let him ask in faith, *nothing wavering*. For he that wavereth is like a wave of the sea driven with the wind and tossed" (James 1:6, emphasis added). We must have faith, and we must be steadfast in that faith.

Whether they were facing teenage struggles or coping with young-adult problems, we determined that every hardship could be handled with faith, and we must not let anything tear down that faith. As we faced things at Emory that tried to destroy our faith, we had friends, family, ministers, and even people we didn't know to build us up. Though the enemy wanted to tear down, God used His people and His Word to build us up. First Peter 1:7 tells us, "That the trial of your faith, being much more precious than of gold that perisheth, though it be tried with fire, might be found unto praise and honour and glory."

Right here in the middle of this test or trial of our faith, in the midst of this lions' den, in the midst of this fiery furnace, God surrounded us with people who believed, people who prayed, people who gave. What a way to build our faith! The Word states, "If ye have faith, and doubt not, ye shall not only do this which is done to the fig tree, but also if ye shall say unto this mountain, Be thou removed, and be thou cast into the sea; it shall be done. And all things, whatsoever ye shall ask in prayer, believing, ye shall receive" (Matthew 21:21–22). We came across this statement online: "Doubt sees the obstacles, but faith sees the way. Doubt sees the darkest night, but faith sees the day!" Remember the promise from a few pages ago about the days ahead not being as dark as what they look like? Sounds like faith talking. Somebody's building. So, Doubt, we have no room for you here! Let's feed our faith, and doubt will starve to death.

Day 25

After a restful night, the nurse woke me up about six a.m., saying, "Mr. Morgan, your fever is going back up." Immediately Mark sent out the word on the blog and to the family to pray that this fever didn't rage again as it had in days past. Within the hour, my fever was heading back down. Praise the Lord! Our next hurdle involved a visit by the Physician's Assistant. She mentioned that the scan on my sinuses on the previous day showed some type of inflammation. She scheduled the ENT (Ear, Nose, and Throat) doctor to do a thorough scan/biopsy of my nasal canal. This would indeed be another setback if it were positive. However, the doctor rolled in her big testing machine. As she began to work, she made it evident that she didn't see anything abnormal. She was quite pleased with everything she saw and assured us that there was no reason to worry. However, she indicated that she would check again on Monday. It's almost as if we take one step at a time and stop on the staircase, praise Him, and continue to the next step. Somehow He continues to give us just enough light and just enough faith to make it to the next step.

During this time, some wonderful friends came to visit with us. They offered their prayers, words of encouragement, and strength. One even brought a homemade pound cake. We enjoyed the fellowship and had another special treat. Brother Ronnie Day, along with his wife, Sister Selena, and his daughter, Sister Ellie, sang one of my favorite songs: "I Still Trust You." It made it so much easier to get through the day knowing someone was sharing the load, whether it was a visit, phone call, or simple message.

The words *just enough* seemed to be the words that stood out. *Just enough* seemed to get us through. First of all, I had *just enough* fever to say I had a fever, *just enough* strength to walk a lap or two around the hall, not enough appetite to eat, but *just enough* appetite to drink my nutrients needed for the day. This reminds me of another great spiritual battle I fought in previous years; I felt the Lord speak to me and say, "Let the Weak say that I am strong" (Joel 3:10). *Just enough!* I might have been weak at that point in the battle, but God was granting … *just enough.*

There are stories in the Bible where just a few fish and loaves were *just enough.* Enough meal for one more cake was *just enough,* a little oil in the house was *just enough*, and one small shepherd boy who went out to fight a huge giant … *just enough!* Little is much when God is in it. There have been times when we have had *just enough* to pay the bill and *just enough* gas to get where we were going. If you find yourself thinking, *I'm just barely getting by*, don't underestimate *just enough*.

Day 26

Day 26 seemed to have no definite beginning because so many up-and-down moments throughout the night kept us from resting for an extended period. As a result, I spent most of the day sleeping and resting. One of the special housekeepers came in to clean the room and asked, "Preacher, how are you today?"

I calmly replied, "Blessed and highly favored, sis. How about you? No need to complain—no matter where I have found myself, I am still blessed!"

No extended testing or blood products were needed. Everything seemed to be so calm, quiet, and peaceful. The only disturbance we had was our old trustworthy and dependable bird dog. He sang and barked more than any other day since I'd been there. The nurses spent as much time nursing the bird dog back to health as they did for me.

The quietness gave us time to reflect on previous days: the hard battles that were behind us already. So many victories. So many prayers answered. We have been brought to a new area on this battlefield. After warriors in a physical battle had fought a long, hard fight, a day of rest was needed for the body to continue. We have thrown Mr. Doubt out of the camp, and we have acquired *just enough* strength to make it possible for a new battle.

While we were waiting for the new "next thing," we couldn't drop our guard, pull off our armor, or get comfortable, because the adversary would be waiting. Though the prayer requests weren't sent out today, we couldn't lay down our spiritual weapons. We wouldn't allow our praise to be quietened down. We would stand guard, hold fast, and keep the victory banner held high. This battle we were engaged in wasn't ours. We were only vessels and tools for the Master's hand.

That day also brought us a visit from a leukemia survivor, Candice, who testified, "If it had not been for the Lord on my side ..." We had more evidence that victory was possible if we stayed the course. We felt like all our friends and family were engaged in this battle with us. Many people sent us stories of victory, testimonies of battles that were hot, tiresome, unexpected, and rigorous! If you find yourself in a battle of your own, Ephesians 6 tells you to gird yourself with the Word, garb yourself with the armor, and grab another soldier by the hand and say, "Fight on. Though this battle may be long, let's endure!" We were ready for the next battle.

CHAPTER 7

IS ANYTHING TOO HARD FOR GOD? (PART 1)

Days 27-31

Day 27

Our days still had no real beginning with the continuation of being up and down all night up to three times per hour. My body sought rest, but people were staying with me, so I couldn't seem to find a place of rest. I had one or two family members who stayed with me continually from my first day there.

Every day at least one family member or friend, someone so close to us that we considered him or her part of our family, stayed in the room with me. The person was determined that I wouldn't fight the battle on my own. He or she was my constant companion on the road to recovery.

Everyone was aware that there would be times when my body

would get weak. They knew there would be times when I wouldn't be able to do anything on my own. It was in those times that I depended on others the most. I needed them to intercede for me when such things happened to me. They knew I would need someone to rely on physically, and they wanted to be there for me when that time came.

You cannot predict things in illnesses like mine. Fighting leukemia isn't black and white. There are a lot of gray areas and uncertainties. You cannot predict when someone will fall sick. You cannot know when he or she will collapse. When you look at a patient, you can never tell whether his or her body will give out as a reaction to his or her medications. A person can become sick in the blink of an eye. And so my family wanted to be there for me, if such a thing happened.

They also knew it was easy for a person to feel discouraged when no one was around to help lift his or her spirits. I became restless sometimes. Part of this had to do with being stuck inside a room and facing the physical unknown, but most of it was because I reacted to some of the medicines I had been given. I stared at the calendar posted on the wall in front of the bed as a reminder of the days of battle we had already come through.

Every day we thanked the Lord for how far we had come. Every day when I was alive, my family and I thanked God for being so kind and merciful. We also counted the anticipated number of days that remained to be fought in this battle. As we prepared ourselves to make it past week four, I felt as though time had stopped. I began to feel restless, for the clock seemed stuck; the days seemed to pass by even more slowly.

The biggest concern that troubled us at that point in our journey was the nasty fever I developed at night. My temperature kept climbing at night. The doctors started running tests on me, trying to find the cause of the fever. When I asked the nurse about the sample cultures, she stated that the group hadn't yet been able to grow anything.

I politely stated, "Any kind of samples or cultures they take— they say they'll grow it out and see what it is. Their farming must be like mine—they don't grow nothing! Because they always say it doesn't show anything!"

The nurse just laughed in response. When she noticed I was uneasy, she explained to me that it was indeed a good thing and that there was nothing for me to worry about. As visitors continued coming in and praying with us, a portion of scripture came to mind. I have it posted in many places at home. It reads, "Let the weak say, I am strong" (Joel 3:10).

There was a definite weakness in my body. However, I knew without a doubt in my mind that I must be strong in determination. Conversations with the visitors who came to see me led to discussions of the need for mighty men of God in our present world, those men who pray and believe with faith that God will work what's impossible.

According to my family, they had heard of individuals' great testimonies, reading our series of blog posts and their declarations of how God strengthened their lives and gave them the courage to say, "I am strong." It's our prayer that all those who read or learn about our story allow God to continue to strengthen their lives and take them to a higher place.

Psalm 91 states, "He that dwelleth in the secret place of the most High shall abide under the shadow of the Almighty." I desire to dwell in the secret place of our Lord so we may abide or live in the shadow of the Almighty. I am reminded that for me to be in the shadow of Him, He must be near us.

The scripture also tells us, "I will never leave thee, nor forsake thee" (Hebrews 13:5). This tells us that no matter what comes our way, God will always be there to guide us and see us through. In this battle, our family has dwelt in the secret place of our Lord, and our friends surrounded us there.

Day 28

Sunday, Day 28, brought in the same nemesis: fever. However, this time it wasn't as bad as other days. The fever, it seemed, was losing its grasp on me. This time the temperature wasn't as high or prolonged as before. We believed prayer was defeating this frequent problem. The other ever-present symptoms were nausea, weakness, and decreased appetite. They told me this was par for the course, but it still was very difficult to get this earthly, physical body to stand, walk, chew food, and even rest.

My son Terry spent this particular day with me, and I would like to use his words to describe it. He wrote an account of what transpired and how it unfolded.

> Daddy resembles a heavyweight fighter in the last rounds of an extended "knockdown, drag out" exhibition. He looks like a warrior who has fought a prolonged, hard battle and become weak and exhausted from it.
>
> He reminds me of what David must have looked like in 2 Samuel 21:15. David and his men were engaged in a great battle against the Philistines, and "David waxed faint." I can picture David so tired that he couldn't even swing his sword or maybe even stand on his own two feet. David was cornered and about to be slain by a giant when Abishai came to David's rescue.
>
> This servant secured David and killed the giant (v. 17). I'm so glad God knows what we need and when we need it. Even though Daddy's physical body is weak, the spiritual man looks quite different— as different as noonday is from midnight and as different as life is from death. We feel assured that this storm in his life shall soon resolve into a deep calm. At this point, we have a renewed sense of hope that all shall be well once again.

At one point, Daddy looked at all of us children and our spouses and said, "I've been 'terror-tized' by all this stuff!" We laughed with him and listened as he explained the fear (terror) each time they hung a new IV drug or asked him to swallow a small cup full of pills.

He fears that it will worsen nausea or make him feel poorer than he already does. Sometimes he just looks at his trusty bird dog (IV pole) and shakes his head. It is then that we watch him settle back and smile, knowing that 2 Timothy 1:7 tells us, "God hath not given us the spirit of fear; but of power, and of love, and of a sound mind."

I remember an instance in my childhood when I was "terror-tized" like Daddy. I was young, maybe four or five years old. Daddy was pastoring at Mt. Olive Holiness Church, and we were living in Miller County, Georgia.

One night, as I was sleeping soundly in my bed, I somehow rolled off onto the floor. To make matters worse, I rolled under my bed while I was still asleep. Then, in the middle of the night, in the pitch-black darkness, I woke up.

I had no idea where I was. Realizing I wasn't in my bed, I reached up. I hit the bottom of my bed frame. *I can't go that way*, I decided. I then reached to the left; I felt there was a way. Thinking I might somehow be under my bed, I concluded that to the right was my way out of this unfamiliar place I had somehow rolled myself into.

So I reached to the right. I hit what I thought was a wall, too. It was actually a sack full of clothes. Panic set in. Wherever I was, I was trapped. Wherever I was, I didn't know the way out! I remember that it was pitch-black darkness that had enveloped me from all sides.

So I did the only thing I knew to do. I began to scream. I screamed one word over and over; I knew that if the right person could hear it, it would make my nightmare stop. If I could be heard, I knew the situation would change immediately. I screamed, "Daaaaadddddddddy!"

Within moments, I saw a light flip on. I heard the rustling of feet, and then I saw those hands, which seemed so huge, gently reaching under my bed. I grabbed onto his hands and latched onto them as though my life depended on them.

And he pulled me out. Daddy came through for me like he always did. I eagerly embraced my father. With tears streaming down my face, I had never been happier to see him than at that moment. In what seemed like my darkest hour, he had rescued me.

He wiped my tears away and held me until I was calm. I knew all I had to do was cry "Abba," "Father," or "Daddy." There have been many times since this night when I have had to call out to him, and his response has always been the same.

So here Daddy is, in his dark place. He has reached up to the left and to the right. The way of escape

seems closed. We have watched him do what he
has taught us for so many years; he is crying to
his father. And it is time for us to come through
for him.

Romans 8:15 says, "But ye have received the Spirit
of adoption, whereby we cry, Abba, Father." As
a family, we are crying out for rescue, and He is
hearing us.

Have you ever been there? Well, you must have, for life is a
series of dark days and dark times. Everyone will face dark days.
Everyone will face fiery trials. If you find yourself in this type of
place, call out to Him. Not only will He change your situation, but
He will also rescue you. We knew God was working to do just that
in this instance. Charles Spurgeon said, "The way to stronger faith
usually lies along the pathway of sorrow." We know these trials are
a necessary part of life.

We also know there is fruit in God's garden that never ripens
until it is bruised. I was feeling bruised. We were looking to be
picked from this trial in the near future. We knew deliverance
was coming soon because we had all been shouting, "Abba, Father,
Daddy!"

Day 29

Day twenty-nine was another one of those days that seemed to
blend in with the days before it because we were up and down
all night—about every fifteen minutes. "Little John" (my name
for Lasix, a powerful diuretic) had been given to me the previous
evening. It certainly helped prove that my kidneys were functioning
normally during this treatment. My fever was less severe, another
blessing of God.

We believe prayers touched heaven for this and for so much more. Both nausea and lack of appetite were very real and predominant. I ate only about a handful of food. The best thing they brought me was an ice-cold Coca-Cola. I drank about three twenty-ounce bottles. After a long, hard swig, I remarked that it was probably worth ninety dollars an ounce.

The rest of the day was exceptionally long and taxing. I struggled for every step. We made two trips around the oncology wing, arm in arm with my son and using a walker. I staggered but pushed through, stretching every ounce of my strength and will.

After the first lap, I became short of breath, but I said, "Let's do one more lap." It was a far cry from the twenty-one laps the medical team wanted daily, but I was thankful for every step, every lap I could do. I declared while we were walking, "God has been good to Junior Morgan!" Even in my time of struggle, I wanted to acknowledge my blessings.

My bed became less comfortable, and sleep came only in short spurts. I knew my family had weak and emotional moments while watching me struggle. I want to paint an accurate picture for you—the ups and the downs of my journey. I want to keep it as realistic as possible. But (and yes, there is always a *but*) we know he who serves the Lord is in far better shape when he is sick than the ungodly when they are full of health and vigor.

Several physicians and PAs came by, and they seemed to spend more time talking to us and answering questions, each leaving us with encouraging words. They said things like, "This is the lowest you will feel physically from this current treatment. You are right on track. Your counts are exactly where we expect and want them." Even in this physically despondent state, we were where we needed to be. God continued to let us know He was still in control, helping us. We have learned that He is always to be found in the thickest parts of the battle.

When my other family members checked their phones, they found a change to my appearance—mostly my head. While taking a shower, I noticed lots of my hair was turning loose. When I got ready for bed, I told my son to "get some clippers!" and I tried to keep the falling hair off my clean sheets. The nurses brought some clippers, and he shaved my head.

I stood and looked in the mirror. I almost didn't recognize the person staring back at me. I thought, *Now I look like a cancer patient. I look like someone battling leukemia.*

But it's amazing what other people see. I've been called a man of God who selflessly lived his life for many years. Others have seen me as a man who loved his family with a love that could come only from God, and they have seen that same God bless us with four healthy children. Still there have been others who think I am a man who is truly blessed by God to have a companion and family dedicated to the Lord. I believe it's safe to say, "God has truly been good to me" and my family. If we are willing to serve Him on the days when we are strong, He will carry us on the days we are weak. We are in His care. And so I say, "Let's do one more lap."

Day 30

It is a common misconception among some modern Christians that this Christian journey should be one of ease. After all, if God is for me, I should face no battles. The way should be plain in front of me, and I should want for nothing. Perhaps they think we shouldn't face difficulties if we are really in the will of God. Maybe we expect the Red Sea to part, the water to gush from the rock, the mountain to be removed from our path, the storm to be calmed, or our children to be delivered simply because we are His children.

In reality, all these things can be done, but they require us to be in the right place at the right time, doing the right thing. Does God really *need* me? He doesn't have to have me; the truth is, *I must have Him!* He can part the Red Sea, deliver the children of Israel, save the lost world, remove every temptation, and provide water without a well, but will I learn anything if He just does it without my submission and *not my permission* (because I will gladly let Him do all that He will) but my *submission*?

These were the next issues we dealt with, facing our greatest battle so far. My body was weak, drained from chemotherapy and other strong medications given to strengthen my immune system. I wasn't able to rest, eat, or even breathe easily. Any of these things can bind a strong man. Pile all of them together, and it became the most intense struggle yet.

When a person is physically worn down, the spirit can easily become the next target and vice versa. Either way, they can feed off each other—that physical man and that spiritual man.

Therefore, we knew we had to battle on both fronts: get the physical man strength and the spirit-man strength. In times like these, we believed this then and still believe it: to whom else can we go but to the Lord?

Only He has the words of eternal life. When He speaks *life*, man must breathe. When He speaks *light*, darkness must go. When He speaks *liberty*, chains must break. When He says, *"Heal,"* sickness must go. When He speaks *peace*, despair has no place.

We have the promises given in God's Word concerning life, liberty, light, healing, and peace. Do they just show up in my mailbox? The Word tells us that the kingdom suffered violence and that the violent took it by force. At this interval in the journey, I required spiritual warfare. For this, my family (and fellow Christians) went to war on their knees.

In 2 Chronicles 20:1, 4, 8–9, 16, 22, the children of Israel faced a battle, in which they desperately needed the Lord's help.

> It came to pass after this also, that the children
> of Moab, and the children of Ammon, and with
> them other beside the Ammonites, came against
> Jehoshaphat to battle. Then there came some
> that told Jehoshaphat, saying, *There cometh a great*

multitude against thee from beyond the sea on this side Syria; and, behold, they be in Hazazontamar, which is Engedi. And Jehoshaphat feared, and set himself to seek the Lord, and proclaimed a fast throughout all Judah ... And Judah *gathered themselves together, to ask help of the Lord:* even out of all the cities of Judah they came to seek the Lord ... *Art not thou our God,* who didst drive out the inhabitants of this land before thy people Israel, and gavest it to the seed of Abraham thy friend forever? ... And they dwelt therein, and have built thee a sanctuary therein for thy name, saying, If, when evil cometh upon us, as the sword, judgment, or pestilence, or famine, *we stand* before this house, and in thy presence, (for thy name is in this house,) *and cry unto thee in our affliction, then thou wilt hear and help ... for we have no might against this great company that cometh against us; neither know we what to do: but our eyes are upon thee.* [They were facing a great battle, but they didn't know how to fight it. They knew only that they had to seek the Lord! The story goes on to say that the man of God gave them instructions.] And he said, hearken ye, all Judah, and ye inhabitants of Jerusalem, and thou king Jehoshaphat, *thus saith the Lord unto you, be not afraid nor dismayed by reason of this great multitude; for the battle is not yours, but God's* ... Tomorrow go ye down against them: behold, they come up by the cliff of Ziz; and ye shall find them at the end of the brook, before the wilderness of Jeruel. *Ye shall not need to fight in this battle: set yourselves, stand ye still, and see the salvation of the Lord with you, O Judah and Jerusalem: fear not, nor be dismayed; tomorrow go out against them: for the Lord will be with you* ... And when he had consulted with the people, he appointed singers unto the Lord, and that should praise the beauty of holiness, as they went out before the army, and to say, Praise the Lord; for his mercy endureth forever ... And when they began to sing and to praise, *the Lord set ambushments against the children of Ammon, Moab, and mount Seir, which were come against Judah; and they were smitten.* (emphasis added)

The children of Israel didn't need to fight physically in the battle, but they had to be in the right place to praise—fully submitted to God. He could have delivered them any way He chose, but they had to do what He asked in full submission. On that day at Emory, God moved when my family and friends got on their knees in obedience, praising Him because He is and worshipping Him because He will get all the glory.

After a month, you would have thought we had faced every situation and circumstance available on this roller-coaster ride leukemia had us on. However, we found this wasn't the case. Day thirty-one proved that more challenges lay ahead.

Day 31

Sherry and Sylena headed to Atlanta to stay with me. On the way to the hospital, Sylena suddenly developed a terrible headache, and they both discerned it was a spiritual attack on her body. It was an attack determined to be an obstacle for them on their way to wage a spiritual battle in my hospital room against the enemy, who was trying to come in with a flood of oppression and despair.

While the rest of the family was praying at home, they prayed immediately for the Lord to move the headache so they could travel on unhindered. Sherry's account provides a unique perspective on the day's events.

Daddy has been extremely weak, unable to eat, unable to walk much, and unable to rest. He has not had a proper night's sleep in weeks. Yesterday, the experimental chemo drug was stopped. He was able to get rid of some of the excess fluid his body was holding on to, and that helped his situation.

Other strong medications were also stopped because the medical team thought those drugs were causing some of these other problems to drag Daddy down in body and spirit. Another doctor came, and Dad got a new mechanism to be a companion to his trusty bird dog. This heart monitor he has named his "purse" because it has to be strapped across his chest when he gets out of bed, like a hobo-strap purse. He keeps funny names for things just like that.

He is scheduled for a breathing treatment ever so often, and those poor souls have to come all the way to his room for him to blow two times in a little contraption. When he sees them coming, he calls them the "breathing musketeers."

His blood numbers looked good, but the recovery process is just moving very slowly, or so it seems. We continued to see the drain and strain on Daddy from all angles, both spiritually and physically. Then we began to recognize another thing that seemed to want to sneak into the room and weigh him down, a kind of darkness or fog that makes it difficult to see clearly. Like a weight that couldn't be lifted, it seemed to drop in a blanket and envelop him.

We grew up way out in the country, so dark at night that you could probably scare yourself if you weren't careful. I am sure everyone reading this can tell we are just basic country people—not fancy theologians. Everything we share we have learned through church and family.

We have grown up on church pews, building friendships of a lifetime with people who are just like us. Real people facing real challenges. We have a choice about how we face those challenges. We can sit down, moan, and groan about our circumstances. Or we can keep living the faith that birthed us, raised us, and has kept us this far.

This isn't the first battle we have faced as a family, but our basis for defense is still the same. Our approach in getting out of it is the same. In every situation and circumstance, what matters first is what God says about it in His Word and second, how we respond to that Word. Third, we face every challenge as a family, and fourth, we trust our brothers and sisters in the church to help us in the time of trouble by holding us up in prayer. It seems simple, but this is the way we live every day.

In the country, we have no streetlights, barely any security lights, and so visitors from town could hardly get accustomed to the darkness. We were acclimated to the dark, so we usually didn't think much about it until we had to spend the night in town.

When we saw it, we were awed. *Wow, so many lights! How do y'all sleep up here?* was my first thought. There seems to be plenty of light here in this city, especially noticeable at night when staring out the hospital window or driving to and from the hospital, seeing the looming buildings and zooming vehicles.

Everything blinking, moving, racing, going, plenty of light—but can we really see, or are these lights merely a distraction? Some are meant to entrap, pulling people into what looks like an exciting place, but actually, those lights hide the ugliness of addictions, where both old and young become slaves to activities that "caught their attention" by the bright lights …

One thing is certain, you can find plenty of light at the hospital and not much actual darkness where you can hopefully sleep. There are examination lights, safety lights, lights on the bird dog (yet to be named), machine lights, elevator indicator lights, vending machine lights, and hundreds of others that are all intended to push out the darkness. In our case, we have lights to push out the physical darkness, but if we are not careful, another darkness attempts to invade our space, and no physical light can chase it away. When this darkness attempted to weigh down not only Daddy's spirit but also ours, we knew it was time to inquire of the Lord.

We remembered the words of the Lord that said He would fight for us, and we also took note of our part: stand still. Standing involves some actual work, especially when all of hell, it seems, is rushing at you, swirling all around, trying to hide and cover up every bit of light you can see. Standing involves not giving up any ground. Keeping the ground that has been given so far, waiting for whatever comes next, but *not* yielding an inch. Standing can be tough. When you stand, you need to believe in what you are standing on and for, and we have promises from God.

Psalm 3 reminds us, "But thou, O Lord, art a shield for me; my glory, and the lifter up of mine head. I cried unto the Lord with my voice, and he heard me out of his holy hill. Selah. I laid me down and slept; I awaked; for the Lord sustained me."

There was the first part of our response, standing on the Word. Next, we determined to stand our ground, praying over Daddy's hospital room and him. The enemy was recognized, and we decided darkness had no place here.

While our family prayed at home, we prayed and begged our friends and church family to pray with us, to bind the darkness threatening to drag him down physically and mentally. We asked them to pray alongside us for him to gain strength, get an appetite, get some rest, and recover. We had a definite battle inside that room, determined to eliminate the darkness trying to invade.

It wasn't an easy or quick task, but eventually word came to us from all around that people were holding us up in prayer. I couldn't help but think of Isaiah 59:19. "So shall they fear the name of the Lord from the west, and his glory from the rising of the sun. When the enemy shall come in like a flood, the Spirit of the Lord shall lift up a standard against him."

Then word trickled down to the southern part of Georgia. Daddy is eating one half of a banana, then later three crackers with cheese, and then an orange. We were almost ready to have a camp meeting. He was able to sit up and talk for over an hour. Then he was able to get up and take a shower. He even asked for chicken nuggets (he didn't eat too many, but he was getting his appetite back).

Praise the Lord! He may not be eating whole meals or running around this hospital or even sleeping all night, but we do thank God for moving the way He has. We are not completely out of the woods, but we know the Lord has got all this under control. We intend to keep standing, to keep doing what He asks us to do. We have placed our trust in the Guide, and we know He shall guide us out of the darkness and toward the light.

We survived another battle, and we were ready to face the next day's challenges, which would surely come. If you are facing battles with an adversary and need overcoming power, you can find your answers in God's Word after surrendering your life to Him. Call on some godly people you know who will *stand* and believe with you.

CHAPTER 8

THE LAST WEEK (DAYS 32–37)

Day 32

In the last week of my stay at Emory, on day thirty-two, the lab test reports indicated that I required potassium and blood products that would hopefully improve my appetite, strength, and rest at night. I was finally able to sleep for over four hours. That was really good, knowing I hadn't slept for much more than one hour at a time without interruptions—either from the bird dog or the constant but necessary monitoring of my medical condition. Consequently, the medical personnel arranged my schedule to prevent interruptions in my night sleep. We believe the Lord provided a way for me to sleep and rest.

The hospital staff was so good to me and my family. They often worked to accommodate us, knowing the stress of the situation could be great. Those days were tough and challenging for us, but we were becoming more familiar with the challenges we would face. When blood products were given, medication to prevent reactions were also given ... and these medications had side effects. Time for another loop on the roller coaster again ... more medicine—less appetite. I was able to eat a few bites (praise the Lord!), and I was able to visit for a while with some visitors from South Georgia. I got up and showered on my own, but we didn't get to walk any laps.

The medical consultants' team visited us and assured us that what many people considered to be the hardest part—the chemo itself—was past us and that we were now in the building-up stage. What we discovered, though, was that this building-up process had its difficulties as well. Whenever I think of building, I recall the biblical story of Nehemiah and how he accomplished the task of rebuilding the walls of Jerusalem.

As mentioned in the book of Nehemiah, he obtained the blessing of the king and took people along with him to help the rebuilding process. One of the first things he did was examine the city and see exactly what needed to be done. Nehemiah secured help from his fellow citizens. They saw the need for the wall—for protection, for strength, for boundaries. Very soon Nehemiah and his people discovered that not everyone was proud Jerusalem would be a protected, thriving place once again. Doubters appeared, and enemies made jokes and threatened. However, Nehemiah was determined in his purpose. "So built we the wall; and all the wall was joined together unto the half thereof: for the people had a mind to work" (Nehemiah 4:6). They had to build with one hand and keep a weapon in the other to fight off their enemies if needed. They were successful because they had the Lord's blessings, and they worked together to accomplish the task.

In our task of rebuilding, we see many parallels here. We had taken notice of what needed to be done to help build me up—rebuild the walls of my city. We had the support and directive from the King—the promise of help and resources. Our brothers and sisters in Christ were fighting for us, beating back the darkness, holding back despair and doubt, helping me to regain the strength to continue my preaching, go to the highways and hedges, and compel lost men and women to be saved.

A united body of Christ (having a mind to work) showed the enemy of our souls that he couldn't have rule or dominion over me or my family. Though some people assumed that the process of recovery would be unproductive for us, we intended to keep fighting and build—a sword in one hand and a trowel in the other. With God as our support, strength, and guiding light, we were able to overcome all hardships. I know we keep mentioning the encouragements, testimonies, scriptures, and songs from our loved ones, but they were a vital part of our building up. It was like each was adding another stone to fortify the wall. That hedge was being built up. When we read and heard that people were praying, we knew they were holding back the darkness of defeat, doubt, and despair.

Day 33

Just when it seemed that things were moving along normally, it was amazing how quickly things changed. We were cruising right along on day thirty-three. After a few hours of rest last night, we were at turtle speed, with less than four bites of breakfast, and starting a day where we thought things would return to normal. I received two units of blood, and I was started on TPN (IV nutrition). Things went normally until late afternoon and early evening. As the bird dog beeped, the doctors, the nurse, and techs came in. Family members changed places as some family members staying in the hospital went home to relax, while others came to attend me. Some young and veteran ministers came to help "build up the wall." Their words of encouragement and prayers were refreshing, and they assured us that people were indeed helping us build and fight on. It is always good to visit with the home folks and with those who are like family.

In the late afternoon, I mentioned to my family to bring a large, poster-sized picture of the grandchildren to put up in the hospital room, since young children couldn't visit patients on my floor. Therefore, they arranged for me to have pictures of grandchildren, aged five to nineteen. The older ones came in, but they all stayed together in the waiting room, not wanting to be separated. Medical personnel continued to allow me to visit the waiting room if I went there while wearing a mask. We had hoped that they would make allowances for them to visit the room. Some nurses claimed my visit would be an extra incentive and strength for me, and I agreed.

Nevertheless, a policy is a policy; precautions and safety are more important in hospitals. My children would print photo books on major holidays, composed of the family photos throughout the year. They brought one of those books to the hospital. As I mentioned about having a big picture of the children, we began to look at the pictures in the book. Again, we were moving at turtle speed, Brenda standing by the bed, turning the pages, and we looked at the pictures together. Within a few minutes, I began to cry, getting more emotional, since I was separated from them at present.

We finished looking at the book, and they put it away. In just a few minutes, the nurse was at our door, wondering what had happened. She said they had called her from downstairs, saying my heart monitor was showing unusual activity. She came to see whether I was turning cartwheels, which was something she had jokingly requested that I do. "No cartwheels," I said. Then I told her we were looking at the grandchildren's pictures, which were the reason for the increase in my heartbeat.

In the afternoon, Becky informed me that the cafeteria was serving fish today. I told her I would like to try some fish pieces, so she hurried down to buy some. Everybody who is closely acquainted with me knows that I *love* fried fish from a certain restaurant near my home. I also prefer home-cooked fried fish, but I just don't eat them from everywhere. When Becky got back to the room, another visitor arrived—one of our cousins, a minister, who came to help build up the wall and push back the darkness. While he stayed with us, I enjoyed his company and ate almost a whole fish filet and part of a hush puppy. (It wasn't South Georgia catfish, but it was so good to be eating something.) Cuz was the nickname we called our cousin, and I talked with him about the Lord and the power of God's Word. I started reading the scriptures we had posted on the wall, with tears filling my eyes. Isaiah 26:4 says, "Trust ye in the Lord for ever: for in the Lord Jehovah is everlasting strength." I said to Kyle, "I believe I am coming out from under this thing; I do."

In a few moments, our nurse came in the room and started working with the bird dog and oxygen stuff. Within a few minutes, one doctor after another began to visit my room. They were looking at oxygen levels and heart rates, ordering lung scans and EKGs stat.

An EKG was completed in a matter of moments, different oxygen methods started, and a chest X-ray was ordered. All that activity took place because the monitoring room downstairs detected a faster heart rate. The EKG was normal since there was nothing serious. That faster heart rate was what we Pentecostals attribute to the Spirit's quickening. It seemed funny to everyone what had happened. It might have caused machines to do strange things today; it sure made them start moving around here really quickly because they thought something was wrong.

On the other hand, it meant something was definitely right. When He said, "Live," man had to *breathe*! That quickening of the Spirit makes the believer feel life. John 6:63 says, "It is the spirit that quickeneth; the flesh profiteth nothing: the words that I speak unto you, they are spirit, and they are life." That wall was being built up, and the Spirit of the Lord was aiding in my defense—pushing back the darkness and despair, showing a big hope for my future.

Day 34

Day 34 began without much sleep from the night before. A severe pain started in my abdomen and wouldn't go away. I had a medical test and X-ray, but the experts didn't get the final results until late. Just before daylight, the pain seemed to recede just enough for us to get a few minutes of rest. The lack of rest didn't stop my improvement, however. Almost everyone who saw me commented on how much better I looked than in previous days. According to my children, I was talking better, feeling better, and looking better. As a matter of fact, when one of my children went down to get breakfast, she found (of all things) fried chicken wings on the breakfast line. How much better does it get than for a preacher to have fried chicken? She brought me some of those to see whether maybe, just maybe, I would feel like eating one or two. She knew I already had some bacon, eggs, and toast on my breakfast tray. When she got back to the room, I said yes; I believed I could eat some of the chicken.

I cleaned off two of the wing bones and was able to sit up and visit my family members and other visitors. All looked happy about the improvements they saw. They asked me if I wanted to walk after a while, and I thought I would walk a lap. We unfastened the bird dog from the wall, and my heart monitor was draped across my shoulder as I shuffled out. I continued to show improvements in my strength and pain level. I was able to put on my new granddaddy do-rag, and Nana put on her do-rag to visit the grandchildren in the waiting area.

The Lord was merciful and kind to each of my children's families, giving them traveling mercy and protection on the trips to and from the hospital. The three-and-a-half- to four-hour trips can be long, hectic, and taxing, especially for those who had to leave the hospital at ten p.m., getting home around two a.m., then going to work early in the morning. But they didn't mind making the trip, even on days when there was spring break traffic, and that made the trip take six hours instead of the usual amount of time. We still thank God for His hand of protection! After all, Psalm 100:5 reminds us, "For the Lord is good; his mercy is everlasting; and his truth endureth to all generations."

While God was working on my behalf at the hospital, He was also providing everything my family needed in surrounding situations as well. Sometimes we are surprised that God performs things we have asked for, and we stand and stare in wonder that the thing is done—that what we have prayed for has come to pass. In Acts 12, we read,

> Herod had killed James, John's brother, and he proceeded further to take Peter also. And when he had apprehended him, *he put him in prison, and delivered him to four quaternions of soldiers to keep him*; intending after Easter to bring him forth to the people. Therefore, Peter was kept in prison: *but prayer was made without ceasing of the church unto God for him*. And when Herod would have brought him forth, the same night Peter was sleeping between two soldiers, bound with two chains: and the keepers before the door kept the prison. And, behold, *the angel of the Lord came upon him, and a light shined in prison: and he smote Peter on the side, and raised him, saying, "Arise up quickly." And his chains fell off from his hands.* The angel proceeded to lead Peter out of prison and to the street. And when Peter came to being himself, he said, *"now I know of a surety, that the Lord hath sent His angel, and hath delivered me out of the hand of Herod,* and from all the expectation of the people of the Jews." And when he had considered the thing, he came to the house of Mary, the mother of John, whose surname was Mark; where many were gathered together

praying. And *as Peter knocked at the gate's door, a damsel came to hearken, named Rhoda. And when she knew Peter's voice, she opened not the gate for gladness, but ran in, and told how Peter stood before the gate.* And they said unto her, "Thou art mad." But she constantly affirmed that it was even so. Then they said, "It is his angel." *But Peter continued knocking: When they had opened the door and saw him, they were astonished. But he,* beckoning unto them with the hand to hold their peace, *declared unto them how the Lord had brought him out of prison. And he said, Go shew these things unto James, and to the brethren. And* he departed and went into another place. Now, as soon as it was day, there was no small stir among the soldiers, what was become of Peter. (emphasis added)

No doubt the people were excited to see Peter. My family and I, too, were excited about the changes we had seen in me for the past couple of days. Late in the afternoon, the heart monitor was eliminated as one of the things I had to carry around—the medical team saw no need for it any longer. Praise the Lord! That was just one of those "chains falling—one less restriction holding me down with the sickness. One by one (or sometimes by twos and threes), we eliminated medicines and treatments I no longer required. Just as prayer was made without ceasing for Peter, we were getting reports of churches, young people, fellowships, youth conferences, and camp meetings fasting and having special prayer times for my family and me.

The enemy may have been seeking to destroy my voice as a watchman on the wall, and he might have planned to have kept me locked me up tight in the inner prison with soldiers guarding me. Nevertheless, the walls couldn't stop the angels or the Spirit of the Lord, and we felt like the light had shone where I was. On that day, I got up and put on my shoes and started walking. We believed in the power of prayer. Matthew 21:22 says, "And all things, whatsoever ye shall ask in prayer, believing, ye shall receive." So ... I went ahead and stepped over those soldiers as they were sleeping. I would step completely out of this "prison" before long.

Day 35

Day thirty-five was tough. As we say on the farm, it was "tougher than a lightard knot or a black gum stump." I battled problems such as fatigue, weakness, decreased appetite, nausea, and abdominal pain. I tried to push through them all, but the weariness of the fight was beginning to tell in my face at times. My family understood that it was normal for a man to feel the pure exhaustion I felt during such an intense fight. *But we do not confuse fatigue with retreat or surrender.*

When you grow up on the farm (and I'm still living on one), there are times when you feel completely exhausted and drained, and you feel like not taking another step. Usually, this occurs in the heat of the day, with a hole digger in one hand and a wooden post in the other. The good thing about a farm is that you can usually find a shade tree to crawl under or a fence to lean against until you catch your breath or what we refer to as "your second wind." At Emory, on the sixth floor, the "heat of the day" was better described as the "heat of the month," it appeared. But God allowed us to rest *just enough* between each serious blow or complication. Whether in prayer or messages, our church friends and church families helped us to catch our "second wind" many times during the last thirty-five days. It was better than a tall glass of sweet, iced tea on a 102-degree, hot summer day. And let us tell you: that is mighty refreshing!

Although I was still waiting on my appetite to resurface, knowing I was getting TPN (IV nutrition) has been a comfort. We joked that the new bag my nurse hung contained "fried catfish." The previous day it had been "steak and potatoes." This was helping, but we know "man shall not live by bread alone, but by every word that proceedeth out of the mouth of God." For this reason, my children have been reading scriptures to me daily.

Sometimes I just started reading aloud one of the numerous encouraging scriptures we had taped around the room. That always seemed to brighten the mood, but then again, we knew there was power in the Word of God—a power that surpassed all the nutrition I could ever receive on a platter in my favorite mill pond restaurant or through an IV bag concocted by the hospital pharmacist. Today Terry reminded me about something that had happened several years ago when we took the youth group from our church to the Little Grand Canyon in Lumpkin, Georgia.

We had twenty to twenty-five teenage boys and girls on this trip, and Terry was probably seventeen. I remember that a group of older teenage boys (seven to eight) wanted to walk through the little canyon and climb out the far side. It was a pretty impressive place. We walked or hiked one to two miles to the canyon's backside and began the climb to the surface. We had to climb about one hundred yards to get out of this huge "pit." At first, it was easy. Then it got tougher, and for the last ten feet (from the top), it was a straight drop.

We found one small pine tree we could use to help us climb out the last ten feet. I helped every young man onto that tree and helped push him to the top of the ledge. Finally, they were all out except one young man and me. I helped him on the tree, and as they reached down to grab his hand, the tree snapped. They pulled the young man up to safety, but this left me ten feet from the top with no way to get out. It looked like I would have to walk all the way back, which meant I would have to spend two more hours just walking around to the starting point. But they didn't want me to go to that trouble, so they suggested a way. What they did may be hard to explain and harder to envision.

About four of the largest boys or young men were asked to hold Terry's legs and lower him over the edge of this small cliff. Terry had to trust them! They lowered him enough so he could lock elbows with me. Terry made sure we had a good hold; then he gave them a sign to pull. Those teenage boys worked together to pull Terry and me to the top of that ledge. We were dirty, but it didn't matter. We were tired, but we were at the top. Ultimately, we were all on top together!

On this day of our journey, it seemed like I was standing just out of reach in a normal situation, wondering how I would get out of this horrible pit. I have tried all my life to help others in similar places get out of terrible situations—not to brag about myself but to help them find the solution to their problems through the Lord. I believe our church family and friends were like those young men, poised at the top of the overhang, praying and working to position my family where they could "lock elbows (or knees)" and literally pull me the rest of the way to the top. I felt weak and needed help. Like David said in Psalm 40:2, "He brought me up also out of an horrible pit, out of the miry clay, and set my feet upon a rock, and established my goings." Together with the church's prayers and God's help, we scaled the last few feet of that steep incline.

Day 36

The next day was the sixth Monday we had been at Emory. The thirty-sixth day was over as I looked at the calendar. We had four attending physicians, multiple physician assistants, numerous nurse practitioners, fellows, and students, countless nurses, and the list went on and on. So many people worked there. So many people filed in and out of my room—there were respiratory therapists, dietitians, palliative care team members, nurse techs, housekeeping and maintenance workers, just to name a few. The most interesting fact is that we got to familiarize ourselves with all of them. Some had traveled there from Puerto Rico, Trinidad, Ethiopia, England, Jamaica, and that far country called "Alabama." Everyone working there was actually from somewhere else (the closest we found was a nurse from LaGrange).

The only constant there seemed to be me, the one everyone revolved around. I don't say that in a way to brag on myself but to let you know that if I hadn't been in that place, none of this would have been going on regarding me. Even my children and their spouses came and went, along with my wife, usually pulling two- to three-night shifts. It has been difficult for them and their families, traveling up and down 1-75 to and from South Georgia every few days. The in-laws left behind had to mostly do double duty.

Every weekend the grandchildren got packed and sat in a separate waiting room for hours, hoping they would get ten minutes to meet me, the man they all called "Granddaddy." Their parents said they loved to see me come into the room. Even though I spoke through a mask and gestured to them with a gown and gloves covering most of my body, they could hear my voice and know this was the same man who would do anything for them. Once the chemo started, I was instructed that I could no longer physically touch them. They learned how to give good "group air hugs." The grand girls mastered blowing kisses to me as well. The hospital policy may have taken away my touch, but a granddaddy's influence could still be felt.

Even though we had tremendous blessings, we also had hardships and difficulties in life. When talking about our previous struggles, nothing compared to what I had faced in the last thirty-six days. We had expected a trial by fire, but this ended up being much more. We expected a struggle, but this had been a war. We knew our faith would be tried but nothing to this magnitude. This sickness and treatment seemed almost unbearable for us.

I discussed with my children how the Romans perfected scourging during Jesus's time. They found that thirty-nine stripes with the cat-o'-nine-tails (a whip with small bone fragments sewn in it) was the most a man could live through. Forty stripes generally killed a man being whipped, so they usually sentenced a man to thirty-nine. They took that man to the brink of death and then stopped, allowing him to live and *try to recover.*

This induction of chemo seemed to follow that same philosophy—take a man right to the brink of death, where his body cannot take one more dose, then stop and let him *try to recover.* I honestly felt like I had been whipped almost to the point of death, but at this point in the struggle, I was starting to recover. The visits, encouraging words sent to me, and the prayers were oil in my wounds, and I knew those would facilitate the healing process.

For the first time, my lab reports about my bone marrow showed improvement. It showed that it started to "rebuild and reproduce." My counts increased fourfold. I still would have a long way to go, but this was such wonderful news to a man who was *trying to recover* after undergoing a tormenting process of pain. Following these tests, a bone marrow biopsy was planned for the next Wednesday, which would further state whether I had reached the goal of *remission.* Nonetheless, we asked for prayers.

The doctor even discussed something encouraging—when I could go home! *If* my blood counts continued to improve and my strength and appetite become appropriate, I *might* go home by the weekend!

Excitement filled the room, and I felt my life returning to normal. We almost sent a runner ahead of us, like the Israeli army used to do, to proclaim that we were recovering and almost headed home. We didn't want to get the cart in front of the horse, but the countdown was on. We knew God had His hands all over our matters, both big and small. We drew strength from Isaiah 41:10. "Fear thou not; for I am with thee: be not dismayed; for I am thy God: I will strengthen thee; yea, I will help thee; yea, I will uphold thee with the right hand of my righteousness."

So now we had more goals:

1. Eat more—I ate three popsicles today.
2. Walk more—I made four laps.
3. Pray more—I felt the Spirit of God shake me today as I called out to Him.

Even though it had been a fierce war from our standpoint, we have had front-row seats as we witnessed what God could do. At that point, we didn't know all the outcomes of this situation. Still, we were assured that He "can do exceeding above all we can ask or think, according to the power that worketh in us" (Ephesians 3:20).

Day 37

I want to let Mark describe the last day at Emory.

> *Tuesday, which was the thirty-seventh day*, was the anticipated day Daddy had been looking for. This day held the words our family had been searching for during these five weeks. The doctor visited my daddy; he seemed to develop a bond with Dr. Khoury quickly. The doctor was kind and motivating; he used terms like *home, family,* and *tomorrow* all in one short sentence. These three terms altogether meant one thing: If Daddy continues doing okay, he would be in South Georgia before sunset on Wednesday. On Monday, Dr. Khoury shared a few things with Daddy that he usually looked for in a patient to release them for home. Today, when Dr. Khoury came to do his rounds, Daddy stood to attention just like he was in boot camp and said, "Good morning, sir!" He meant he was heading

south, even if it meant chewing on an energy bar, which tasted like cardboard. As it turned out, Dr. Khoury had expressed concern about the calorie consumption Daddy needed to recover his stamina. Daddy explored his mind to determine what he could eat that wouldn't make him sick rather than build his strength. Therefore, he requested a bowl of chicken noodle soup to sip on. The nurse tech brought it to him after warming it up, and he started eating. While taking this high-energy soup, he visualized that he saw Shamba (his name for Mama) and Nashville's lights in the bottom of the bowl, and he meant he was going to finish. After spending countless dollars running all over northeast Atlanta, trying to find something to reactivate his taste buds, a two-dollar can of Campbell's Chicken Noodle Soup, located down the road at the local grocery market, did the job. He said this was the only thing that tasted the same.

Watching day thirty-seven has reminded us of a story found in Ezekiel 37, the story of the valley of dry bones. Today, as Daddy was trying to come to grips and handle what has happened here for the last thirty-six days, it became evident that the Spirit began to quicken his body. His feeble, frail body gained strength by the second with each "Praise the Lord" and "Hallelujah." It seemed as if the very breath of God was breathing life into his dry and weak bones. Ezekiel 37 starts out by stating, "The hand of the Lord was on me." Countless times over the past few weeks, our God has breathed life into our situation. This question rings over and over in my mind: "Son of Man, can these bones live?" Looking with our carnal eyes, many would say there is no hope ... it was full of dead men's bones ... Thank God for life!

The hand of the Lord was upon me and carried me out in the spirit of the Lord, and set me down amid the valley which was full of bones. It caused me to pass by them around about: and, behold; there were very many in the open valley; and, lo, they were very dry. And he said unto me, Son of man, can these bones live? And I answered, O Lord God, thou knowest. Again he said unto me, Prophesy upon these bones, and say unto them, O ye dry bones, hear the word of the Lord. Thus saith the Lord God unto these bones; Behold, I will cause breath to enter into you, and ye shall live: And I will lay sinews upon you and will bring up flesh upon you, and cover you with skin, and put breath in you, and ye shall live, and ye shall know that I am the Lord. So I prophesied as I was commanded: and as I prophesied, there was a noise, and behold a shaking, and the bones came together, bone to his bone. And when I beheld, lo, the sinews and the flesh came up upon them, and the skin covered them above: but there was no breath in them. Then said he unto me, Prophesy unto the wind, prophesy, son of man, and say to the wind, Thus saith the Lord God; Come from the four winds, O breath, and breathe upon this slain, that they may live. So I prophesied as he commanded me, and the breath came into them, and they lived and stood up upon their feet, an exceeding great army. Then he said unto me, Son of man, these bones are the whole house of Israel: behold, they say, Our bones are dried, and our hope is lost: we are cut off for our parts. Therefore, prophesy and say unto them, Thus saith the Lord God; Behold, O my people, I will open your graves, and cause you to come up out of your graves, and bring you into the land of Israel. And ye shall know that I am the Lord when I have opened your graves, O my people, and brought you up out of your graves. And shall put my spirit in you, and ye shall live, and I shall place you in your own land: then shall ye know that I the Lord have spoken it, and performed it, saith the Lord.

Ezekiel 37 is a message of hope. So often we could hear that soft voice speaking "life" as blood counts came together and strength was granted. Thank God for life! Multiple times today, Daddy said, "Thank God for the Holy Ghost!" In this vision, the valley was full of dead men's bones. During this time, when a battle was fought, the victorious soldiers would strip the valuables from the slain and leave their enemies bodies unburied. Sometimes skeletons remained for years afterward until beasts came and scattered the bones. Our enemy wanted to leave us in this valley lifeless. He wanted to leave Harvey Morgan's bones in this valley of death and despair, but God breathed life!

Again, Ezekiel 37 is a message of *hope*. A message that God's Spirit can bring life to any situation and any soul, no matter how hopeless and dead they may be. Let God breathe life into your dry and dead situation, whether it be a valley of health issues, marriage relationships, finances, or discouragement.

I recollected the words of the song by the Horn family.

I just came into a valley I cannot believe.
My heart began to ache with pain for all the sights I've seen.
There were bones lying everywhere of people that I knew.
I began to cry and wonder Lord what did they do?
Then I went on in the valley, the casualties were high.
There had been no struggle because Satan had won the fight.
Then I heard the devil call to me they're gonna find you next,
but I *turned and looked at him* and this is what I said. …
You won't find my bones down in this valley I am coming out!
I've seen too many fall around me but that don't make me doubt.
The devil will try to bring me down, but I will not give in
'Cause all you'll find down in this valley
are the *prints of where I've been*! (emphasis added)

CHAPTER 9

HOMECOMING

Day 38

Certainly day thirty-eight, Wednesday, March 19, 2014, will be in our hearts forever! We got up that morning with anticipation so thick, you could feel it. We heard that the ones at home were excited, but the ones with me in Atlanta were doubly excited (if that's possible). The doctor had mentioned the possibility yesterday of going home, and I grabbed "ahold to it!" I might have wrestled with it all night, but I wasn't going to let it go.

When the doctor peeked in the room, I was ready for him. Nothing was going to stand in the way of that vehicle heading south. The staff started getting the paperwork ready, and the text messages and phone calls started flying in. I know Verizon had to have experienced an overload, because my poor telephone could hardly keep up. Family members back home started coordinating the food and fellowship for the family, because we knew it would be a celebration.

Some of our family-like hospital staff walked us down to the vehicle, and we were glad to have made friends. We know without a doubt that God placed individuals in that unit to take care of me and my family. The doctors, nurses, and techs were somehow part of His grand design, even down to the air musketeers, who had to stop and read the scriptures posted in our room and comment on how much concern and love were demonstrated and felt there. One even proclaimed, "There is nothing more powerful than Jesus!" It was amazing to see the change come over them when they saw the words of the Lord, knowing it was okay to speak them, use them, and believe them. As great as that part had been, it was time to leave this part of the journey and start back toward home.

Balloons, banners, posters, and food for all the Morgans (and some Watsons, who didn't want to miss the homecoming) were assembled on Highway 135 in Nashville, Georgia. Terry's wife, Leigh, and our son-in-law, Doodle Bug, helped coordinate those balloons, banners, posters, and food. They made sure the freezer was stocked with Klondike Bars, because I learned those were something I enjoyed eating while in the hospital.

Instead of "Can you hear me now?" which is the usual cell phone message when talking, we were getting, "Where are y'all now?" They wanted to know how much time they had before they would see us pulling up in the yard. The family posted pictures online of what was waiting at home so our friends could see our excitement. They had balloons and signs leading up to the driveway, with most of the family standing in the yard. The grandkids were either in the back of the truck or being held there, while holding onto balloons and a big sign welcoming me home and welcoming those who were bringing me.

Finally, the vehicle arrived with the horn blowing. Everyone was clapping and cheering, and they let the balloons go. When the vehicle stopped out by the road, I got out, hugged Brenda, and then hugged everyone standing there. It was most definitely one of the most moving moments I have ever experienced. All my family could say when I hugged them was "Praise the Lord!"

My reply was, "He is a mighty God. That's the reason we are here today!" So many tears, but these were happy tears.

After sitting and talking for a while, we ate supper, which had been donated by a business (Tip Top) in Douglas, Georgia. When they learned what we were celebrating, they wouldn't accept payment for the food. We received the same treatment when we tried to pay for the huge banner the kids were holding when I first arrived in the yard. The blessings just kept coming!

My family would still have to be overly cautious around me, keeping loads of hand sanitizer and face masks for company. Medically, they told me my immune system wasn't fully recovered (but so much better so quickly), and I was supposed to avoid crowded places for several days. My heart was so glad, glad, glad to be home! Whatever the restrictions or limitations on my travel, I was willing to agree to almost anything. No doubt God had plans for a man He told, "Live!"

One of the verses my children put up on the wall in my hospital room for me to read when I woke wake and had the strength to focus on was found in Mark 2. The passage is about the man brought to Jesus who was so sick that his friends had to lower him through the roof because there were so many in the house to see Jesus. When Jesus told the man to get up and take up his bed, things began to happen. "And immediately he arose, took up the bed, and went forth before them all; insomuch that they were all amazed, and glorified God, saying, We never saw it on this fashion." It has taken all my family and friends to bring me to the Lord.

I believe they expected to see me get up at any minute, going down the hall and proclaiming the greatness of our God. They finally got to witness this very thing. Suddenly, strength came into my body (results of the prayers of the saints), and gradually it increased so much that I was increasing in strength through the day instead of decreasing. In talking with the doctor during this week, the man with the medical credentials said, "Your blood work doesn't look like the blood work of a man with leukemia."

Yes, we were all amazed because we hadn't seen healing in this fashion! Apparently, some of them had not seen it like that either, because no one expected us to go home that soon—especially a man of my age. Since the previous day, I gained strength to eat, walk, pray, testify, and proclaim the goodness of the Lord. When God says, "Live," you have to expect to live! All throughout the day, I shed tears while thinking about the goodness of the Lord.

We brought home the rollaway bed my family purchased while we were at Emory so two family members could stay comfortably (as long as one person stayed on the hospital-issued couch) with me during those rough nights when fever would rage or pain would zap my strength. My family calls it the "hospital bed," and we refer to it as the bed we took up, going forth from the hospital, proclaiming victory in the name of Jesus. One thing is for sure: none of my family members wanted to miss that first church service I was going to attend in the next few days. You talk about rejoicing; there has been some around the Morgan household, but when we enter His courts—look for some praise. We intended to make His praise glorious.

Day 39

It was so good to wake up at home for the first time in over six weeks. I didn't sleep much. I was accustomed to someone coming into my room for blood work every few hours, but I felt like I rested better while being in my own bed. On our family farm, I had a Great Pyrenees, which stayed with my dairy cows. From the first night I was back home, he made himself a bed under the window outside my bedroom, which had a lamp and shined almost continually. I think somehow he knew I had been sick. If I got up during the night and moved around the house, I could hear him outside, moving around as well, outside the window where any lights suddenly turned on.

The first full day home continued to proceed with a few bumps, but whoever expected smooth sailing just because we left Atlanta and Emory University Hospital had slightly misread the forecast. There was some weakness, nausea, and anxiety when we arrived home, but "home" even made those more bearable. My appetite was slowly increasing. The old nemesis, fever, was low grade, off and on. The family was being extremely cautious about using antibacterial, antiviral, and antimicrobial lotions, gels, and sprays to ward off things we couldn't even see. It was much like staying "prayed up" to try to keep the enemy off your back.

In the wonderful jubilation of our homecoming day, we recharged our tired bodies, spirits, and minds. With all my family gathered around my great room at home, I was almost like a kid, grinning from ear to ear about simple things that most everyone takes for granted—like the feel of our favorite recliner, the close intimacy of gathering around a dining room table, children constantly scurrying around and giggling, the taste of good well water, the loudness of family, and the quietness of the country—just to name a few. I was like a sponge absorbing every word, and my emotions were tender and true.

I had never realized that the one thing I had taken for granted was my time with my family. We sometimes think things that are unmovable and deeply rooted are just expected to last and be present—indefinitely. During busy lives, we forget there is a God-ordained cycle to life, and we need to appreciate everything good in our lives *right now, at this moment.* I guess what I'm saying is, tell someone today what he or she means to you. Don't wait. Share with someone the message of hope and salvation today. Don't wait. Life can change from calm to chaos in an instant, from peacefulness to perplexity with one phone call.

So many people, some known and others we weren't familiar with, have commented on the faith of our family through this great trial. We felt we were no different from any other family. We fought doubt, discouragement, fatigue, emotions, tempers, and so forth just like everyone else. We were ordinary men and women. We aren't great orators, scholars, kings, or saints. We are schoolteachers and administrators, health professionals and business managers, preachers and singers, husbands and wives—just like you. We *all* (you and I) have this great resource of strength in Christ Jesus, and it is amazing to see the results when we *choose* to trust this resource.

Storms come, sometimes suddenly and quickly. They might pounce from every side. We feel surrounded and can hardly breathe. If you are in one, you know what I mean. If you are not in one today, you know as well as we do that one may be in tomorrow's forecast. But our testimony is that He has proved Himself so many times to us, not only in those thirty-nine days but in *all our lives*. So I believe I'll testify one more time, sing one more verse, say one more prayer, speak one more encouraging word, because He is worth trusting. Our question is, how about you? Be assured that He is closer than you can even imagine.

Even though it seemed that Thursday revealed just how weak and fragile my body had become, both Friday and Saturday of my homecoming week proved to be days when strength began to show up in greater spurts. I started moving very slowly but deliberately, determined to be all that I could be, in this place we refer to as home. I, along with my family, had uneasy moments where we weren't sure how to respond or react to fever, nausea, or simple fatigue. In the previous weeks, we had our wonderful nursing staff to rely on for the answers. At this point, we had to look over the home instructions we'd been given and hope we were doing the right thing.

A big difference we noted was with my body temperature. I would stay cold, usually wrapped up in a jacket or robe over my regular day clothes. When people came out to see me, I was wrapped up tight in my recliner, while Brenda was on the other side of the room in her recliner with a personal fan blowing. The air conditioner in the house wouldn't get much of a workout during that summer. In communicating with the nurses since we left

Emory, they told us that one characteristic of patients like me was the fact that we would always be cold. That was okay with us, of course, especially knowing this was nothing unusual—just another situation with which we would learn to cope.

As we sat around the house and farm for a couple of days, one of the best things I noticed was the increasing strength and resolve. Every time I said yes to a suggested food or attempted to go outside just to stroll up the driveway, I saw that as a way God was increasing strength minute by minute, hour by hour. My family had been trying to help do some home maintenance chores here at home, and I couldn't simply sit still and let the workers take care of those things. I had to make the effort to see about what was being done.

In the meantime, neighbors dropped in just to see for themselves how I was doing. In addition, I had numerous phone calls and answered questions about how I was really doing, and I was so glad to know people were concerned enough to check on me personally.

During all this hanging around at home, I developed a taste for popsicles, which my family found very funny. I had never been much of a popsicle person, but for some reason, I began to like them fairly good, which was great, according to the grandchildren. After all, if Granddaddy was eating popsicles, surely it was okay for them to have one, then another, and yet another. Some of the family tried to spend the night with us because they had become so accustomed to staying with us at the hospital. For weeks, one of the children stayed with us every night but one. We assured them that I would be okay and that their mom could take care of me.

People from the community and our church friends, who lived within driving distance, were so good about visiting us and asking what they could do to help. One of the neighboring families brought in a huge meal for our family to enjoy during the first few days I was recovering. Other neighbors and friends also dropped by to see whether we needed financial assistance or help with anything around home.

Days 40–41

Next came days forty and forty-one, with day forty being the day when it was prophesied that I would find strength. Amazingly, my family watched me enjoy the blessings of the Lord, heard me speak of the might of our God, and shared my desire to do more for God in the days to come. Ezekiel 16:6 had served as our motto since day one, when we began this long journey. The days ahead will provide more opportunities to show how we will continue to hold fast to the promises of God and *live*!

One of the best things about home was the ability to sit in my recliner. It had comfortably suited me for several years, and the family knows it as my chair. If anyone is sitting there when I come in, he or she vacates it because it is known as mine, even now. From my earliest days of arriving home from Emory, if I woke in my bed during the night and couldn't sleep, I stumbled into the living room on my walker, found the recliner, and rested there until daybreak.

Brenda returned to VSU to continue teaching her classes, and I was at home from about 7:15 to 4:30 each day. Most days found me in my recliner, gaining strength and soaking up the atmosphere of home. My appetite still wasn't fantastic, and one of the older ladies in the community heard I was having some issues with eating or not really wanting to eat much. She made a big pot of homemade chicken and dumplings and sent them to me. It was awesome; I continued to gain nourishment and strength. I had left home at around 200 pounds, with my normal hair parted on the side and combed as usual. When I returned home, I was about 140 pounds, bald, feeble, and frail. When I saw myself in the mirror, I knew it was just a physical skeleton on the man I had been before going to Emory. However, when God says, "Live," we must live.

A week after coming home, I reported back to the Winship Cancer Institute for an additional bone marrow test. That test showed I was in remission; *healed* is the word we used. Even though we had participated in a trial treatment while at Emory, I was unable to complete the treatment there because it made me so sick. We had different visitors who dropped by the house on various days, but especially the weekend. They wanted to see for themselves that I was really doing well.

I normally had two to three doctor's appointments per week, because I was sent back to Dr. Shah at Tifton Oncology for further testing/treatment. Usually Becky or one of the other children drove me to my appointments for blood tests and treatments the doctors thought I needed, even though they had declared I was in remission. Blood levels remained constant, but I still didn't attend church services for several weeks due to being cautious about my immune system. I found that Dairy Queen milkshakes were also particularly good at helping me gain bodily strength and improve my appetite. I didn't usually say much while riding. There was a lot to think about.

CHAPTER 10

WHAT WE HAVE LEARNED

The six weeks of time we spent in E6 definitely served as a reality check, but that time was also part of our spiritual growth. As a family, we learned many things about faith, focus, and service during these last few weeks. We learned that no one is immune to great sickness or trouble. Matthew 5:45 tells us, "For he maketh his sun to rise on the evil and on the good, and sendeth rain on the just and on the unjust." Just because you are a born-again Christian, that doesn't exempt you from facing the circumstances of life. You will have problems and sicknesses, just like other men. All things may not turn out the way we expect them to go. What sets us apart from the world is that we trust that God has a bigger plan than what we can see *at the moment*. We know nothing is too hard for God, and He will help us get through whatever we are facing as long as we are trusting Him.

We realized that keeping the Word of the Lord in front of you as much as possible can help you move along the road to recovery.

We know His Word is powerful and alive and can speak to our hearts and lives. John 15:7 reveals, "If ye abide in me, and my words abide in you, ye shall ask what ye will, and it shall be done unto you." Having the reminders of those faith scriptures where you can see them will help you build your faith. You can write the scriptures down on posters, index cards, or a whiteboard. You should try to write them down wherever you can easily see them. Doing so can encourage you to continue in your faith. Motivational speakers and self-help gurus encourage people to write motivational sayings on mirrors or paste them in prominent places where they can be seen. So placing the never-changing Word of the Lord would be that much better! Several people who visited us, including hospital workers, commented on the faith evident by the Word being displayed visibly where we could read it daily. It also served as a witness to others who entered the room that faith was important to us.

Another realization that has proved to be the most amazing to us is how much strength we could gain from the words of those around us. Words always have an impact regardless of the medium used to convey them—whether they are sent by phone or computer, in a text, in comments on a social media post or blog, or in letters and cards. Phone calls also proved to be a powerful encouragement. Our friends sent us words that brought much comfort during the most trying time in our lives. These words were another source of strength during long days and nights. They instilled determination on days when we felt like we weren't making much progress. Even now, we can read back over their words and still feel the love, support, and reassurance encompass us again.

In addition, we learned how important it is to reach out to others in time of need, especially during extensive hospital stays. The family of a sick person is under such strain both emotionally and physically. During extensive hospital stays, a visit from a loved one or friends can bring them a small ray of happiness. Any words you could offer to ease anxiety or encourage them are greatly appreciated. Not only words but actions can also provide support to families who are in a great crisis. We had people who brought baskets of fruit and snacks, homemade cakes, and other goodies. They also brought vending machine coins, dollar bills, and other monetary donations whenever they came to visit. Paying for parking passes for people to stay at the hospital was also a lovely gesture. Coloring books, activity books, and simple games for kids to play while they are waiting could be something you might provide to a family in distress to help them out. Another possibility you could provide for people are power strips for cell phone or iPad chargers, which are necessary devices for people as they provide updates for those who are interested. Every deed committed with good intentions is worth more than gold in this world. Whatever it takes to ease the family in distress could help bring a small sense of joy in their worlds.

We learned that we need each other. Family and friends' visits are extremely helpful, especially when people are mindful of the sick person and don't stress him or her with extremely long visits. People who drive every mile—whether near or far— or go out of their way to get to the hospital or long-term care facility significantly impact both the sick person and his or her family members. People definitely need each other! Also, it can be very stressful for only one person to stay in the hospital with a sick person facing a life-threatening illness. In our situation, we learned that two people should stay to encourage each other. This way one person doesn't become physically and emotionally worn down. It's easy for the enemy of our souls to bring in discouragement, fear, and doubt when a person is weak in body and spirit. Hospital stays are stressful and can wear down even the strongest of people.

Through these experiences, we learned that home is a very sacred place and should be loved, honored, and protected. I used to think that home was a place you could go to when you couldn't go anywhere else. However, you never know when you might not have the privilege of being home whenever you want to go. Every day, I looked forward to the time when I could return home, and it bolstered my hope that my health could be regained. I longed for the time when I could sit in my recliner with my family gathered all around me. Recovering in the comfort of home was an experience that definitely moved me farther along the journey to good health. Even though I received top-quality care (and Emory did the best they could), being home allowed me to rest better. It allowed me to sit out on the front porch swing or ride on the Ranger to the ponds in the fields and enjoy the scenery of nature.

This time of sickness and healing directly impacted my family in ways I might not fully be aware of, so I asked them to write a short response about that time.

From Becky's Perspective

The strength and resolve I saw in Daddy during this sickness is something I will never forget. If you had told me on the last Sunday that Daddy was at Emory but that he would be home by the next Sunday, I would have been sitting in the doubter's seat for sure. He was so sick the previous weekend, but we know God touched him so he would be able to come home. Brother Kyle had spoken previously about his strength renewal in the coming days, and the darkness Brother Nathan referred to had been revealed.

This taking hold of life (based on Ezekiel 16:6) reminds me of the story of Jacob in Genesis 45. Jacob's sons had gone into Egypt because of the famine, and while there, their brother Joseph recognized them. He wanted them to get Jacob and bring him back to Egypt. "And they went up out of Egypt, and came into the land of Canaan unto Jacob their father. And told him, saying, Joseph is yet alive, and he is governor over all the land of Egypt. And Jacob's heart fainted, for he believed them not. And they told him all the words of Joseph, which he had said unto them: and when he saw the wagons which Joseph had sent to carry him, *the spirit of Jacob their father revived*" (emphasis added).

We have seen our father's spirit revived, especially since the day he came home, with an increase every day. Those ministering angels have been quite busy this week, bringing strength, power, life, and more endurance. He can visit more, walk more, eat more, sit more, and stand more.

I remember a specific time after Daddy had been home for several days. I had spoken to him on the phone, and he sounded so weak and frail. I allowed doubt and questions to fill my mind about whether he was really going to be back to his old self or not. I was part of a family group text where we offered updates, support, and encouragement to each other. In this text group, I mentioned that things didn't seem to be looking good at all. Daddy seemed so weak and sounded so frail.

Immediately, my family encouraged me to hold on to the promises of God—that He never wavers on His promises. He had said, "Live!" Therefore, things *would* get better. They told me we had come too far to doubt now. It was so easy to just go on what I could see at the present time. Fear and doubt tried their best to discourage me, but when the enemy came in like a flood, the Spirit of the Lord raised up a standard against him. I remember falling to my knees and crying in my living room floor, once again declaring the victory God had promised my family.

While I was sitting by Daddy's recliner on Father's Day, he read a card I had given him. I told him I sure didn't like seeing him so weak and frail. He looked at me and said with resolve, "It ain't gonna always be like this!" I will never forget that statement. That has been one of the truths we have witnessed from that time of sickness. To look at him now, you would never know he had come that near to death and escaped to live!

In every trial and dark time in my life since that time, I think of those words: *"It ain't gonna always be like this!"* There will be victory if you have a promise from the Lord. One of my favorite scriptures has always been Micah 7:8. "Rejoice not against me, O mine enemy: when I fall, I shall arise; when I sit in darkness, the Lord shall be a light unto me." There may be times where your family members are discouraged during times of great sickness or distress; when that happens, encourage, uplift, and inspire them to continue trusting in the Lord. *It ain't gonna always be like this!*

From Mark's Perspective

I remember starting my day off like any other day on February 10, 2014, the day before the nineteenth wedding anniversary for me and Sylena. I was at Liberty Faith Christian Academy that morning when I received a call that told us the doctor had requested that Daddy head to Emory. Immediately I went and told Sylena and got the girls out of class and told them what was happening. We went to the chaplain of the school and had prayer before leaving, not knowing that God had a miracle in the making.

We headed to see Daddy and decide on what needed to happen. Terry and I took Daddy to Emory, and this is where it all began. We worked as a family to ensure that Daddy had someone around the clock, staying with him to help with whatever he needed. We began making contact with individuals, asking for prayer, and we held on to the verse of scripture the Lord had spoken to Daddy only hours before. Ezekiel 16:6 says, "And when I passed by thee, and saw thee polluted in thine own blood, I said unto thee when thou wast in thy blood, Live; yea, I said unto thee when thou wast in thy blood, Live."

Prayer was the focus of this time because we were always taught the power of prayer. We knew that if we could believe, Daddy could experience healing, and it could be a testimony to people to build their faith. One day we were talking with the doctor and were expressing concern; the doctor alluded to the fact that we couldn't compare our experience with another patient because the dynamics in this room were different from those in the next room. What she meant by that was that she saw the faith each of us had and felt the prayers of our friends as they passed through the doors. This had an impression on many doctors and nurses, and they watched the Lord begin to work.

One night late, we received a call to rush to the hospital because Daddy was experiencing a bad night from the chemotherapy. When we arrived, the nurse said she had placed Daddy on an ice blanket, trying to get his fever down, and she said, "We have done all we can do." It was at this point that we knew if we didn't see a miracle, we had heard the last sermon preached from Daddy. We began praying and believing that God would move. At one point, Sylena and Sherry got the oil bottle and anointed every corner of that room, rebuking every evil spirit. We saw a complete turnaround, and the healing process began.

The experience we gained from Emory is one that will never leave my mind. I watched and saw how God took a terrible situation and used it for His glory. My children were able to see God's hand at work and watch how He was able to do all things.

From Sherry's Perspective

As I reflect over the week of the diagnosis, many emotions resurface, and I have a couple of points I would like to share. I recall Terry putting us on a four-way call with Becky, Mark, and me. He informed us that while the diagnosis was bleak, we could still beat it. I remember fear/sadness wanting to rise, but faith took over and took the lead. Our faith had been built on the foundation that with God *anything* was possible. We had seen many miracles in our lifetime that had built our faith. My dad was a firm believer in healing. He had prayed for many people to be healed; now it was our turn to pray for him.

Our next step was making plans for the next couple of months. We all met at Mom and Dad's home. Dad had already heard from the Lord when we arrived. He began telling us the scripture the Lord had laid on his heart. My mind began to wander. What was the "formula" or "requirements" for a miracle? I wasn't sure, but I intended to do everything to bombard heaven in the request for one. I believe prayer, fasting, faith, worship, and the power of the Word are important in receiving from the Lord. My girls were ten and twelve during this time. Every Bible in our house was turned to Ezekiel 16:6 and placed in various places in our home. Any time we walked by one, we read or quoted it. I stressed the importance of "believing" it—not just reciting it or reading it. We hid this Word in our hearts! Throughout the next few months, we continued this, and it became the basis of our faith. We took this scripture and many others to Emory Hospital and posted them on the walls for all who entered to read and believe. Scriptures of healing and faith were reminders of what God could and would do. We needed these reminders when Dad's fever got so high and the nurses had exhausted all their efforts and limits to reduce it.

While the Word of God was evident and an important part of our petition for a miracle, we also were in constant prayer, as was the church. I recall when the fever raged to 104.9; the nurse had exhausted her limits. She looked at me and said, "I don't know what else to do." We immediately began praying and even sent out the "text alert" for prayer. In about fifteen minutes, we watched the fever start coming down. I listened closely and watched the nurse. I also heard her in the corner praying. She checked the temperature every two to three minutes to see whether it had come down. Not only did the Lord prove His power to us, but He proved it to her as well. What a witness of His power!

I also recall another time when a spirit of "death and depression" was present in the room. It seemed like every bit of information we got back in South Georgia wasn't good news. Sylena and I were scheduled to stay the night. We decided to take a bottle of oil with us and pray over the room. We prepared our hearts for the task during the drive up. When we arrived, we informed the family that we were there and to start praying. We began anointing every window, door, crevice, and so forth with oil and took authority over every spirit of depression and sickness. Luke 10:19 says "Behold I give unto you power to tread on serpents and scorpions, *and over all the power of the enemy*" (emphasis added). I do believe this was a turning point for us. Sometimes we have to fight for our miracle. It wasn't but a few hours later that Dad was asking for a banana and an orange to eat after he hadn't eaten in several days. We cut up the banana, and he put it in ice chips and ate it.

Previously, I mentioned the "text alert." Let me explain further. The support we had was amazing. It was as if it came in layers. I feel like we had a layer of family support for Mom. Then we had a huge layer of support under us from friends, coworkers, church friends, and then people we didn't even know. This group seemed to grow daily as the word of Dad's sickness was spread from church to church and state to state. The "church" held us up through prayers, phone calls, visits, blog posts, and so forth. They were there when the "emergency text alerts" went out. They were consistent, when the blog posts were written, to read and respond. Every response was welcomed and needed. All this provided the layer of support needed to keep our faith strong and our spirits encouraged. God's people are amazing. Many even came with messages of hope, songs of healing, and words of comfort. I encourage you to reach out to your church and get involved. Your church can be the constant encourager in the hard times and crises that will battle you throughout life.

While my heart is so full while recalling these events, I hope they encourage you and reassure you that there is nothing God cannot do. At times, especially with a "bleak diagnosis," we may feel like somehow God's hands are tied, or He is so far up in the sky that He isn't concerned about us. Psalm 120:1 says, "In my distress I cried unto the Lord, and he heard me." These scriptures can be found all throughout the Word of Him hearing the cries of His people. Cry out to Him today, surround yourself with people of faith, and watch God do the impossible.

CHAPTER 11

THE AFTERMATH

I wanted to share my story because it is my personal testimony of how the Lord moved for me when no one else could help me. This story shows there is strength in unity and togetherness when faith is built on faith. When people come together, there is power in unity, power that moves mountains, fills valleys, and crosses deserts. Faith calls things done, even though they seem undone. Faith moved the Red Sea, opened the rock for water to gush out for over a million people and their livestock, conquered nations, and defeated enemies. Faith declared hope when there was no hope, healed lepers, opened blinded eyes, caused the dead to live again and children to be restored to their parents. Faith made me whole.

We received some very encouraging messages during the time I was at Emory. These messages appeared on our family's blog and really encouraged us as we faced some dark, dark days. We were in awe that these words not only gave us strength but also uplifted others, who visited our blog in hope of encouraging my family and me. Here are some of the messages we collected:

Bro. Junior and Morgan family, y'all have been great friends to for many years. I'm not a writer, but I am a reader. I look forward to reading these updates and comments every day. This morning the song on my mind is "What a Mighty God We Serve." I'd like to share a portion of my morning devotions. When the foundations are shaking, remember that God is still in control. His power isn't diminished by any turn of events. Nothing happens without His knowledge and permission. You're in our prayers and thoughts all the day long. We love y'all. RR & SR

I love reading the good news! You are constantly in our thoughts and prayers. I can't help but believe that *great* testimonies are going to come from all this. He's working a mighty wonder, and once on the other side of all of this, you will surely look back in amazement of all that God was doing. He has His hands in this matter and He's doing something great!

While praying for you last night, my mind went back to all the years you served as pastor at Liberty Faith, and I couldn't help but wonder where my little family might be today without a pastor who preached the truth to us and cared for us so sincerely. A pastor who was concerned about us and, when we would start to drift off course, would set us straight again. You've spent your life encouraging and praying for others, and now we are doing the same for you. We are standing with you in this battle, and we are believing with you for a great miracle from our God. Keep on keeping on! Thanks be to God, who causes us to triumph always in every place.

We love you and are praying! DC & JC

We come to this blog to find out how God is working in Bro. Morgan's life and always leave so encouraged! What a mighty army of people God has to stand behind one of their own in time of trouble. Keep looking up; the mountains are full of God's heavenly host. Parkview Calvary Holiness Church is still praying for a full recovery. Much love to you all. JS & CS

One of our nurses, Gladys, even shared the blog with her family and friends back home in Puerto Rico. We had visitors to the website from Germany, too. We had people praying in various parts of the world.

As I read the blog, I thought of these verses:

Psalm 24:8, 10—"Who is this King of glory? The Lord strong and mighty, the Lord mighty in battle … Who is this King of glory? The Lord of hosts, he is the king of glory."

He has shown Himself to be strong and mighty many times. Praise His name!

Continuing to pray and believe on your behalf.

I know that He is able and He will carry you through this dark time.

AG

Daddy, at my work station here in the office, I have a calendar Leigh made especially for me. It has an important photo next to each month. She will pick a special photo we have from the past year and make the calendar for me every December. Today I flipped the calendar from February to March (I'm a few days behind!), and there was a reminder to me of everything for which you stand. My March photo is one of you standing in Bro. Fred Smith's pond, baptizing Emma. There in the calm waters you stand like a tree, holding her gently, helping her proclaim to everyone there that she was a new creature in Christ. I had to go in my office, overcome with emotion. I know I've told you before, but thank you for being the best man I know. We still have one more girl to baptize (Ava), and I look forward to watching you help her proclaim the same. I love you. TM

Terry, thanks for the tears this morning. Love that comment. Reminded me of the time he baptized me at Kinard Bridge. It was one of those times when we had about twenty wanting to be baptized. I can just see it: his left hand on my back and his right hand pointed toward heaven. His voice ringing out strong: "In humble obedience to thy command, I baptize this, my brother, in the name of the Father, the Son, and the Holy Ghost." Oh, the memories we made over the years when he was our pastor. I truly think he is one of the best men who has ever walked this earth. Brother Junior, keep the faith. People are praying daily. Love y'all, and can't wait to hear you preach again. JD

Much, much prayer going up for Bro. Morgan on this Sabbath day. This morning our pastor talked about an ordinary man doing extraordinary deeds … about how wonderful it must have been to live during Jesus's time on earth and witness His mighty deeds. My mind kept going to Bro. Morgan and his family as they pray for and witness these extraordinary deeds on the sixth floor at Emory University right now. We will all continue to pray for strength and wellness … believing that our Lord will provide. Love y'all. AL

I am reminded of Moses in the fight with Amalek. He stood on the top of the hill with the rod in his hand. As long as Moses held up his hand, Israel prevailed, but when he let down his hand, Amalek prevailed. But eventually Moses hands were heavy. That's when his friends came to his aid. They got him a chair (rock) to sit on and got on either side of him and held those hands *up*. Bro. Junior's hands are heavy, so first of all, his family and next his friends are coming to his side to hold those hands up. My prayer is you will be strengthened today, first of all, spiritually ("He giveth power to the faint; and to them that have no might he increaseth strength."). And secondly physically, that this enemy that has raged against you will be defeated. Your friends are praying. Be encouraged. FS & JS

I don't even know how to tell you all how much I look forward to hearing the good news of what God Almighty Himself is doing personally for you, Bro. Junior, and also what it in turn is doing for the family! What a way to start out Sunday morning … Hallelujah! He's taking the shackles off one by one and getting us ready to all dance/rejoice in His name! We love you guys and are praying for you daily! So thankful for everything the Lord is doing, whether it be the small things or the bigger things … Each and every one of them is a great and mighty thing, and He deserves the glory and honor and is so very worthy to be praised. Love and prayers! GC

I remember that trip to the Little Grand Canyon like it was yesterday! Thanks for this encouraging post. Joseph and I were talking about this not long ago. It was pretty scary, but we made it through and have a good story! Brother JR has made it through many battles, and with this battle, he will have another story to reach the lost with! Love ya'll and continue to pray daily for our dear friends, the Morgan family. CH

When we read back over some of the messages from our friends and acquaintances, they fill us with joy all over again to know God had an army of believers who were ready to fight for us against this sickness. Through the prayers of the people and His Word, He proved that when He speaks, He means just what He said. The scripture given to me—Ezekiel 16:6—continued to be our anchor. God said, "Live!"

After I returned home, I continued to hear from others how my sickness and recovery had influenced the lives of those I knew personally and others who had simply heard my testimony but had never met me. We have written testimonies from people (specifically given to us to share) who were directly impacted. It had been suggested to me that I add these testimonies to our story to show that we don't travel through life alone, especially on this

Christian journey—that others are watching and that others can be helped in ways we don't even realize. These messages aren't meant to bring glory or honor to me but to give praise and recognition to God for His abundant blessings on my life.

The Reverend Edsel Young, moderator of our church association, wrote,

> Brother Jr Morgan didn't begin to be an inspiration after his episode of being healed, he was one previously. But it's very likely that because of that bout with cancer, a greater fire of God was kindled within. God decided and declared His work wasn't over, only changing gears and accelerating. God didn't have to allow this that He might draw him closer but rather to show him greater glory. His resounding message to me is to do something for the sake of the gospel, make a difference in the world's mission field, which surrounds you. How can words describe his character, convey his demeanor, or value his worth? We use endearing terms as friend, peer, and even brother. Even language has its own limits as to what Brother Morgan has meant to so many. Thank you, my brother, for your contributions to our generation and your timely responses to desperate and wayward souls.

The Reverend Freddie Stone sent the following words:

> When I first heard Brother Junior Morgan had leukemia, we didn't want to believe it, yet we knew it was true. Bro. Junior wasn't just a person we knew but a close friend of our family. All through our ministry, we had been in church and rode

many miles together, preached, been in revivals, and saw the power of God. We have been through many storms together and knew God was able to bring him through this one. Of all the storms, this was probably the darkest by far. We were holding to Ezekiel 16, in which God passed by Israel and saw them polluted in their own blood and said, "Live." He saw Bro. Junior in his sickness, and He would have mercy and say, "Live." God brought him to the very door of death and raised him up for a testimony, and his family has testified of the miracle-working power of God. We saw the word of faith produce the work of faith. God raised him up, and he has pastored again and is now preaching in various churches. We thank God for what he did in his life for the glory of God.

Pastor Ervin Lewis sent us this letter:

It gives me great pleasure to write a portion about such a great miracle. I consider it an honor to be asked.

Brother Morgan was at my church in January just a few weeks before he was diagnosed. When I found out he was sick, it broke my heart. Every morning I would get up and check the blog for updates. It was there that I read about the scripture in Ezekiel that God had given him. I know there were ups and downs, good days and bad days.

One day, not long after I found out, I felt the need to go see Bro. Junior. My wife and I left one Friday after lunch and drove to Atlanta. The next morning we went to the hospital to see him. I have to say it was hard watching a man of his caliber dealing with everything that was going on. But God's Word was true, and His promises prevailed over sickness.

Sometime later, we were eating out after church at Steak 'n Shake. I was seated next to Brother Morgan; he began talking to me about his experience. He said there had been days when he could feel himself literally slipping out of bed and dying. He said there were times when he had just wanted to go home and die. But he held onto the promise, and God came through just like He said.

I believe the following January, he and sister Morgan were back at our church, preaching another revival. God will bless the faithful. God will honor the prayers of the praying man such as Bro. Morgan. Thank God for healing! Thank God for His promises, and thank God for mercy!

Pastor John Sewell declared,

Hebrews 11:1—"Now Faith is the substance of things hoped for, the evidence of things not seen." Brother Junior Morgan's sickness with AML called on us as a church and individuals to stand on this verse. Lessons of faith are mostly from personal experience. Prayers, confidence, testimonies, and statements were seasoned by faith in God's healing power during those days. In hindsight, my faith was increased while observing the miracle God had performed in Brother Morgan. Brother

Morgan's miracle has and continues to serve as a testimony and help to many people.

Tony McBrayer, secretary for Pineview Holiness Baptist Church, wrote the following letter about my miracle:

> Harvey Junior Morgan (Bro. Junior to us) became our pastor at Pineview Holiness Baptist Church in November 2013. Four short months later, he was diagnosed with acute myeloid leukemia (AML) and given two months to live. Though stunned by the news, strangely we didn't feel hopeless or devastated. When we had voted Bro. Junior in as pastor, it was evident that it was God's will. We couldn't accept that he would be taken away from us so quickly. Bro. Junior received his diagnosis on Tuesday morning. The following day, at our Wednesday night church service, God reinforced our feelings of refusal to accept the verdict of this disease by visiting with us in a mighty way.
>
> After one choir song, Frances McBrayer felt we should anoint our associate pastor, Bro. John Sewell, on behalf of Bro. Junior. As we gathered around the altar and began to pray, the Spirit of the Lord settled down in our midst in such a tremendous way. In fact, Frances, who was seventy-five years old at the time and has been in countless church services as the daughter of a holiness preacher, said she had never felt the Spirit as strong as she did that night. Deacon Troy McBrayer felt in his heart after this mighty move of God that Bro. Morgan would be back as our pastor. Faye McBrayer Roberts reminded us that Bro. Junior had proclaimed in

a recent service that Pineview Church was about to see a miracle, and she added, "Little did he know that he was going to be that miracle." The Spirit was so strong in confirming to us that he was going to be healed that I felt led to take a victory lap around the inside of the church as a symbol of claiming the healing that was on its way. Knowing that Bro. Junior was leaning on Ezekiel 16:6, reading the family's expressions of faith on the blog, and hearing about the scriptures on the wall of his room and the effect they were having on the hospital staff all served to encourage us at Pineview and strengthened us in Christ. When we received negative reports about Bro. Junior's condition and the devil tried to make us doubt the healing we had been promised, we pointed him back to this Wednesday night service, and our faith and belief were renewed.

Joy Jackson Clark, one of the excellent nurses from Emory at that time, said she still stresses the need of patients to see or be with their families as much as possible during their sickness and treatments. She uses this example to support her claim:

Mr. Morgan wasn't feeling well, and normally he could make it outside to visit the grandbabies. Not this time. We also had him on "telley" (they monitored his heart on another floor). Family had left but surprised him with a picture album. I went to check on him and found him resting. A few minutes after leaving his room, I got a call from the floor monitoring his heart that something was going on … I needed to go check on him; his heart was beating much faster than normal. I walked back in to find that the reason his heart was racing was from the happiness of going through pictures of his family. The picture album sat in his lap!

A great friend of the family, Jean Carol Ruis, sent us these encouraging words:

> Harvey Morgan, Jr., or simply "Bro. Junior" to our family, is a dynamic Pentecostal preacher whom I have known for approximately fifty years. He is considered a "hero of the faith" by many including me. Thus, upon receiving the shocking news that Bro. Junior had been diagnosed with acute myeloid leukemia (AML), the realization of putting faith to the test became apparent. Did we really believe that "the effectual fervent prayer of a righteous man availeth much," as stated in the Bible and taught our entire lives? Was this too hard for God? It was time to "rally the troops" and pray to almighty God, our healer, on Bro. Junior's behalf.

> During Bro. Junior's illness, his devoted family surrounded him, reading scriptures, praying for his healing, and earnestly requesting prayers from everyone they could. Throughout the entire ordeal, Bro. Junior's faith he had preached about to thousands never seemed to waver. He had many days of pain and suffering, putting his faith to the test. A petition for healing of this devoted man was diligently prayed for by countless friends, acquaintances, family, and especially by Bro. Junior himself when he was able, with confidence it would be answered. Just as promised in God's holy Word, by divine intervention from our God and

surpassing all human understanding, Bro. Junior was healed from AML. Praise God! Rejoicing was heard throughout the country. Along with his family and Bro. Junior, I thank God to this day for the miracle of healing. What a mighty God we serve!

Here are some thoughts from Pastor Greg Roberts concerning my miracle:

In the Gospel of St. John, chapter 9, we find a very strange story told of a man who was blind from his birth. Nothing strange about an individual being born blind, but verses 2–3 are what make this story one of the most striking encounters where Bible readers are brought face-to-face with a very imposing question Jesus's disciples asked Him. "Master, who did sin, this man, or his parents that he was born blind?" Then one of the most complex answers that falls on man's ears concerning this blind man is, "Neither hath this man sinned, nor his parents: but that the works of God should be made manifest in him." What a complex answer for such a sincere, imposing question! Are you telling us this man had to go through life up to this point blind just so the works of God should be made manifest in him? Is it possible that some people are chosen to go through some awful situations, painful encounters, or dreadful sicknesses just so the works of God should be manifested through these people?

Could that have been the case with Bro. Junior Morgan? A man of God, a man of prayer and fasting, a friend to the brokenhearted, a man of good health. One day he stepped into the chosen timeframe of God and was diagnosed with acute myeloid leukemia—as one chosen by God for this dreadful disease? Just so God could work His works in him so we could be stronger believers? Yes, it is possible, and I believe that is what happened. Look what we all learned from his faith through this sickness.

The difference between the miracle of the man in John chapter 9 and Bro. Morgan's miracle is how quickly, by obeying a command to go and wash in the pool of Siloam, he received his healing. Bro. Morgan's miracle wasn't as quick or simple as going to a pool of water to wash and come back healed. His healing was over a period of time—time so more and more people could witness the miraculous miracle of the powerful manifesting works of God. All of us who were involved in praying, fasting, watching, and waiting learned so much from Bro. Morgan and God's people from far and near. Churchgoers and non-churchgoers were influenced as we saw God use this man of God in this sickness.

We all know God is able and willing to speak the word of healing at any time for the miracle to happen, but let us fasten our eyes a moment on Bro. Morgan. After all, it was he who had to go through this trial—possibly just for us, for us to have more faith, for us to trust God when hardship knocks us down, when the enemy attacks our lives, when the devil ambushes us with his arsenal of doubt, fear, anxiety, or sickness. Yes, it was possibly just for us!

A man who was so sick he was hardly able to hold his head up—he would whisper words of encouragement and faith to keep believing God for His help—not only for himself but also for our family, our churches, and our nation ... A man whom others would go visit to encourage him would leave with a word from heaven themselves ... A man whom God used to minister to others, even while fighting this awful disease and being so sick from it ... Oh, what faith, what hope, what strength we were taught by God through this man of God and his faith during the time of his fight to live.

I met Bro. Morgan when I was a young evangelist. I have known him for many years. We have preached for each other and traveled to preach in far countries together. He became my pastor when I moved from Alabama to Georgia. He has helped me many times with his faith, words of wisdom, and ministry. God brought him out of his sickness like He did the children of Israel—with a high hand! Praise God!

I am so sorry he had to face this trauma of sickness for the betterment of our lives in the kingdom of God. Thank God and him for all we learned from this! It will forever be in our hearts how he entered *and* exited this battle, preparing us for any attack on our lives. Thank you, Bro. Morgan, for the faith, trust, and love of God you have helped impart into me and my family's lives. You are greatly loved and appreciated by the Roberts family.

Evangelist Silas (Doodle Bug) Carver, our son-in-law, sent us these words:

> Just as the disciples were honored and blessed to be able to walk with Christ and see His mighty miracles firsthand, I was honored and blessed to be able to see God's mighty hand at work through Bro Morgan's journey.
>
> There were many miracles along the journey besides the great miracle of his healing. I recall one day when he was going to need a blood transfusion, but when the blood test came back before doing the transfusion, his count had gone up to the equivalent of a pint of blood. There were many more times when God moved mightily.
>
> One thing that really stands out in my mind is that when Bro. Morgan and the family got the awful news of AML, he told us to go somewhere and leave him alone for fifteen to twenty minutes while he prayed. After I returned and talked with him, he said God had told him he could come on home if he wanted to, but if he stayed, He would use him some more. Thank God for a man who isn't just concerned about himself but has such a burden for others that he would choose to stay and go through what he did to be able to keep preaching the gospel of Jesus Christ!
>
> Our God is a Healer!

All these testimonies are humbling and make me weep, confirming my belief that God healed me for a purpose bigger than I knew. He had promised my church a great miracle, and I believe my healing was part of this miracle. When my strength was recovered, our church launched a tremendous outreach ministry called "Peanut Butter & Jesus" in Tifton, Georgia. I had been praying about an outreach program and found two vans in a neighboring town that had been used for several years with a local ministry. I could tell those vans weren't being used at that time, and I was able to contact people who owned them. Their volunteer base was no longer in operation, so they agreed to donate the vans to us. We started this ministry in Tifton on September 23, 2017, by distributing approximately 140 lunch bags. With our team of volunteers, we currently deliver as many as 1,750 bags to hungry children every Saturday! We feel blessed that God has allowed us to be part of a simple but powerful ministry.

This ministry feeds needy or hungry children and disabled elderly people from the community by delivering a sack lunch to their door on Saturdays and other times as the need arises. In each bag, we place a peanut butter and jelly sandwich, a snack, a drink, and a kid-friendly gospel tract. At the time of this writing, PB&J-Tifton has delivered over two hundred thousand sack lunches with two hundred thousand tracts in the local community, and we now have four vans instead of two. Please visit this website to learn more about this 501(c)3 organization: https://peanutbutterjesus.org/.

God's plans are so much bigger than what we can usually see. It has been my desire to be used by the Lord, and I want my story to be something that will possibly change your life as well. If you are facing a great sickness or personal crisis, others may be watching you and your faith as you go through that experience. No matter what circumstance you may be facing as a believer, you can win your battles through faith in the Lord. We look at these battles as ours, but God's Word declares that they belong to Him. If you will call out to Him, He can provide what you need. Isaiah 41:17 says, "When the poor and needy seek water, and there is none, and their tongue faileth for thirst, I the Lord will hear them, I the God of Israel will not forsake them."

To the unbeliever, we hope our healing experience will help you to understand that God is real and that He stands by His Word. If He is calling you to become His child, He offers salvation for the soul, healing for the body, and keeping power for the soul. All you have to do is trust, believe, and have faith in Him. You must acknowledge Jesus as the way to the Father and recognize that He loves you and that He died on the cross for your sins (John 3:16). We hope you will receive the knowledge of Christ and become aware that you need His grace. You can determine today to become the born-again child of God and have life more abundant. Please reach out to us if we can provide any additional information you need.

Every story of how lives have been touched by ours during this time of sickness has been the oil of healing poured in our wounds. If you have a testimony of how this great battle has affected you, please share it with us, with your friends, and with your local church. After all, you are made an overcomer by the word of your testimony and by the blood of the Lamb. We have been amazed by some of the stories we have heard so far. We share them all with tears and thanksgiving.

If you have had faith renewed, have discovered a relationship with the Lord, or have simply regained a second wind, we would love to hear about it. Please send us an e-mail at harveymorgan1011@gmail.com or write to us at the following:

God Said Live!
c/o Harvey J. Morgan
P. O. Box 57
Lakeland, GA 31635

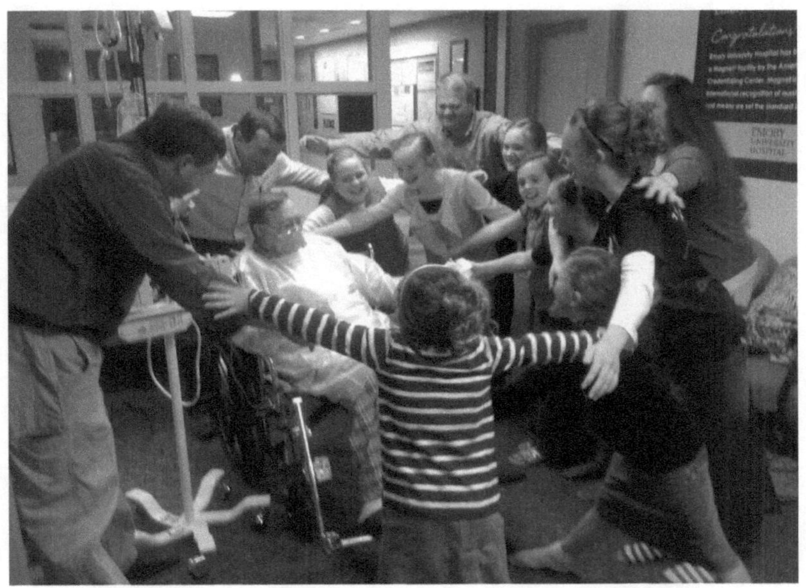

*When I visited the grandchildren in the waiting room, they learned
to give air hugs (due to my compromised immune system).*

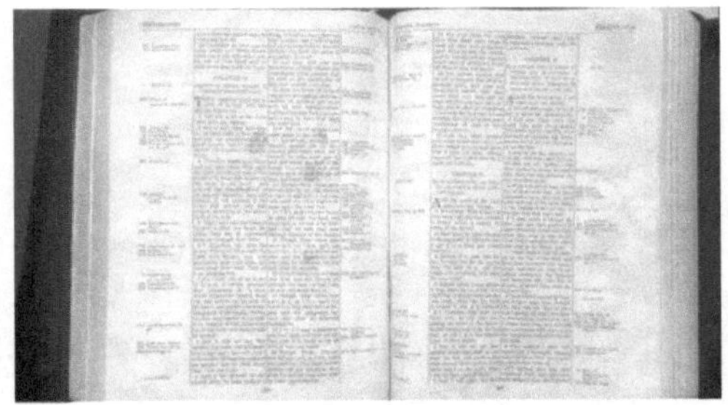

*When my family returned from praying in the chapel after
hearing about treatment options, they found my Bible open,
where I had been praying. I was ready to go or to stay.*

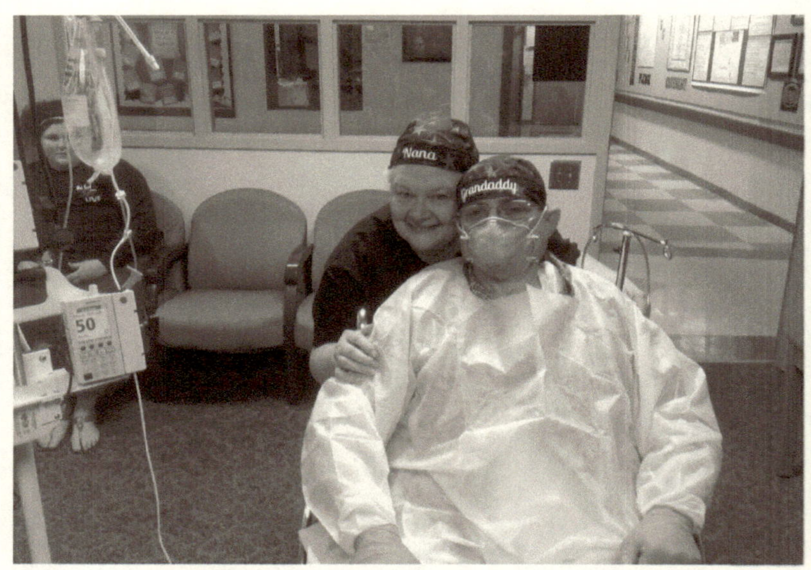

After losing my hair, my sister Doris sent do-rags for both me and Brenda. I wore this when I went to visit family in the waiting room.

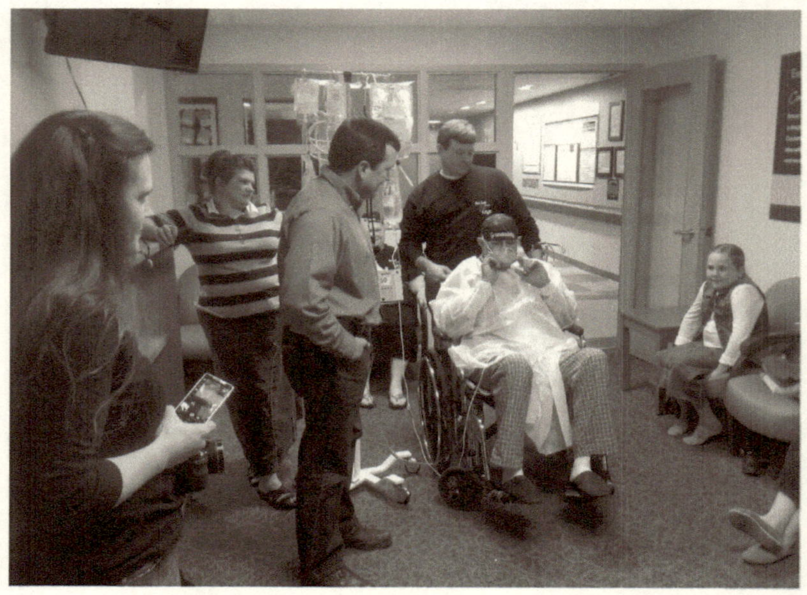

All four of my children spent weekends in and around Emory while treatment was administered. Their children mostly stayed in the waiting room.

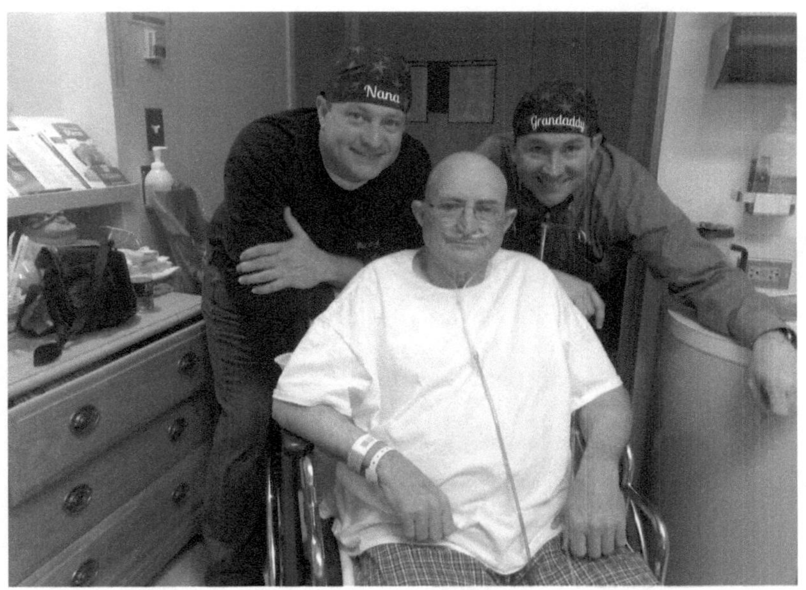

One of my first pictures without hair... I am beginning to look like a cancer patient.

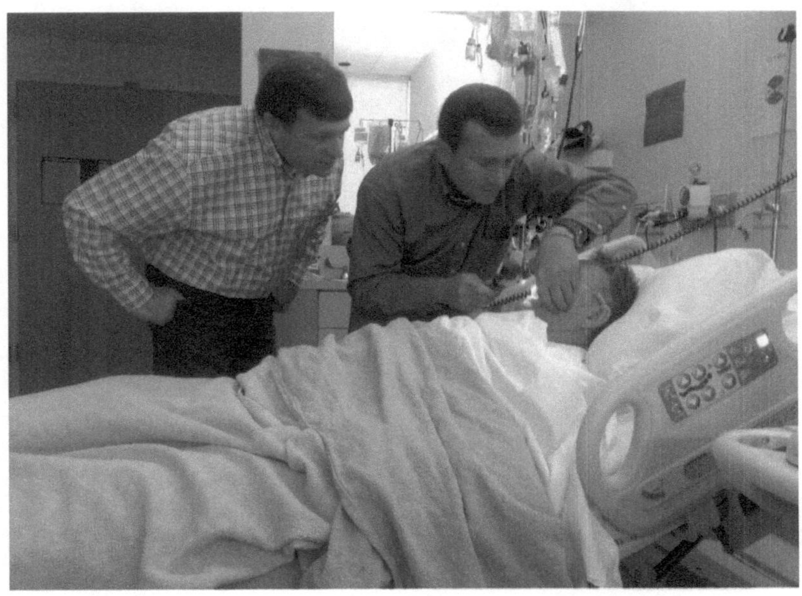

One of the side effects of chemo was sores developing in my mouth.

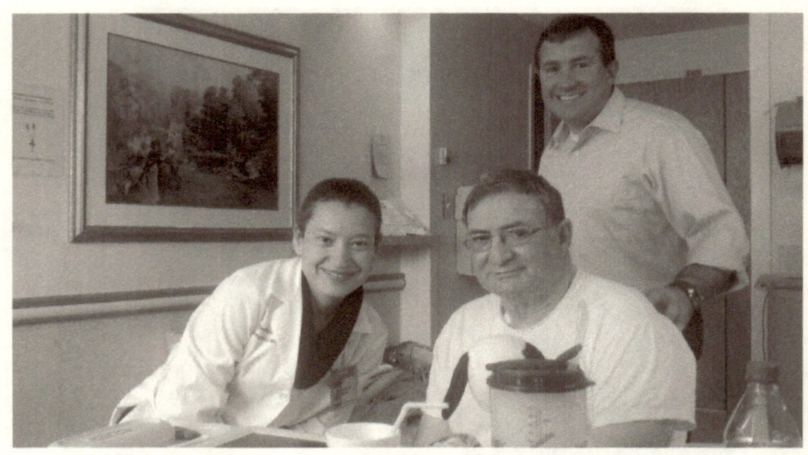

Dr. Martha Arellano from the Winship Emory Cancer Institute was part of our treatment team.

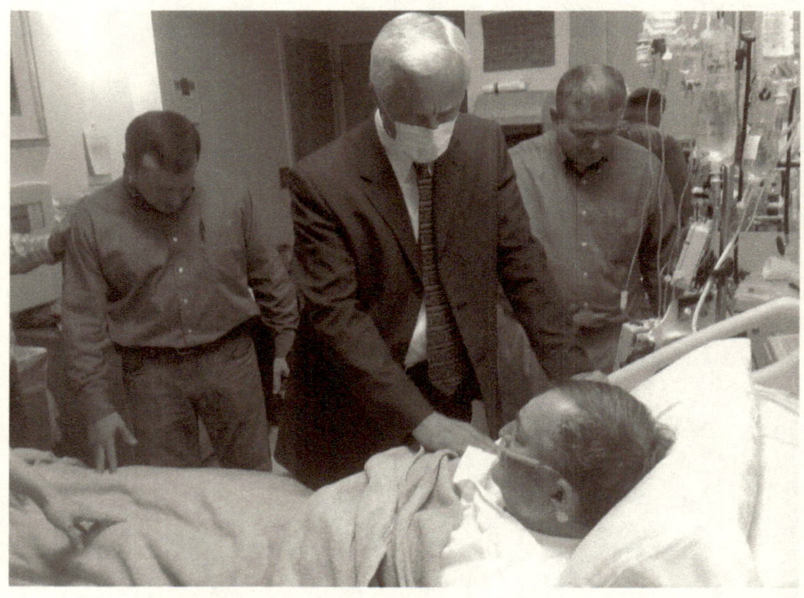

Bro. Edsel Young, Superintendent for Holiness Baptist Association, was one of the many ministers who visited and prayed with us.

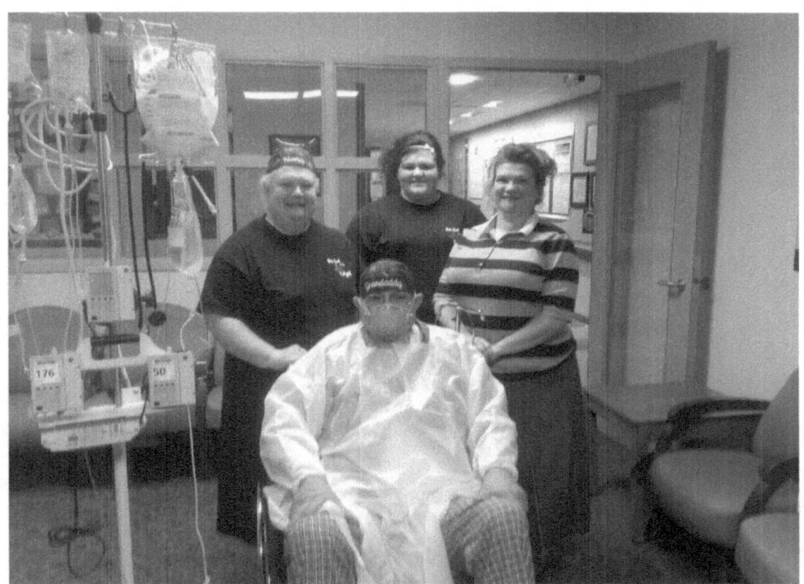

Part of my family and "the birddog" (IV pole), which was my constant companion.

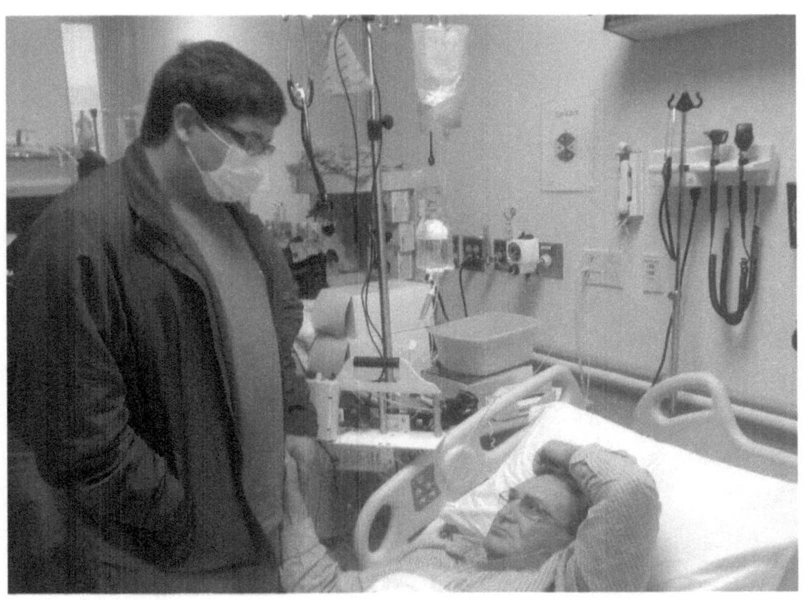

My only grandson, Gage, as we visited during my hospital stay.

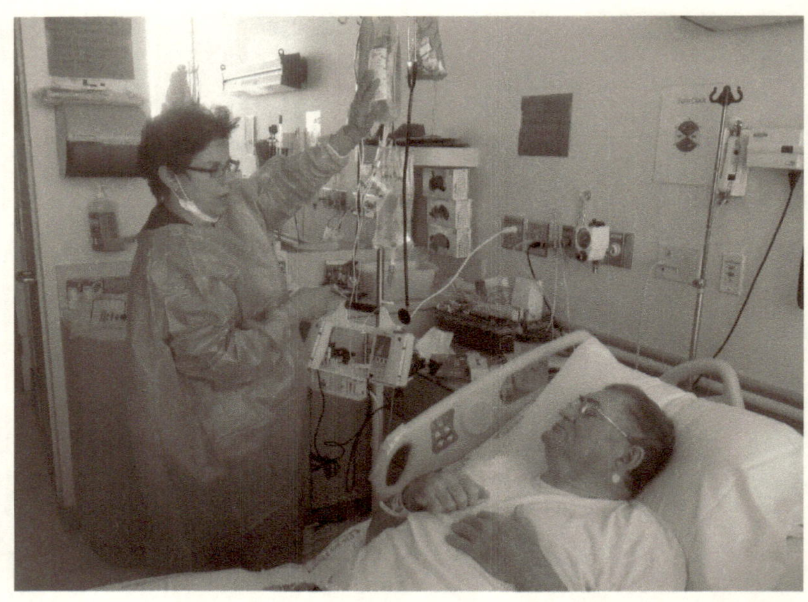

One of our special nurses, Gladys Jusino, who became a good friend to our family.

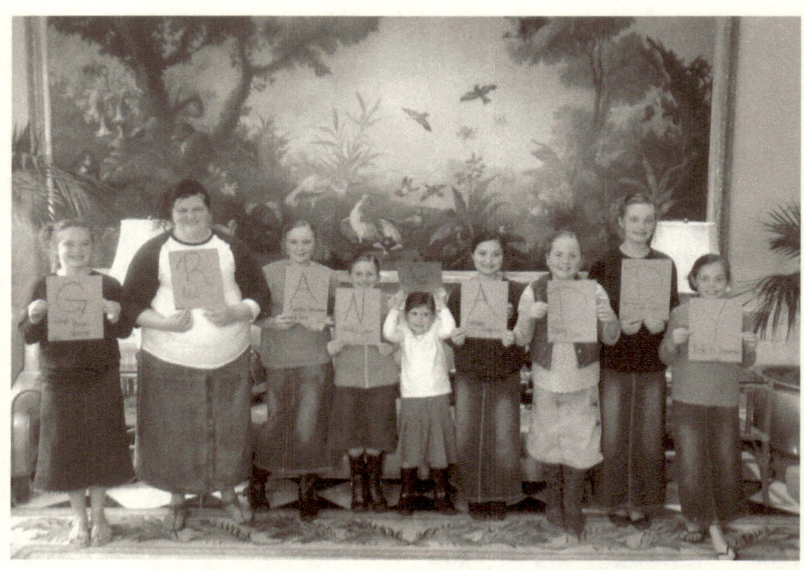

*The grandchildren liked to plan special "programs" for me to try
and cheer me up. Here they spelled out Grandaddy and came up
with a word that described me for each letter of my name.*

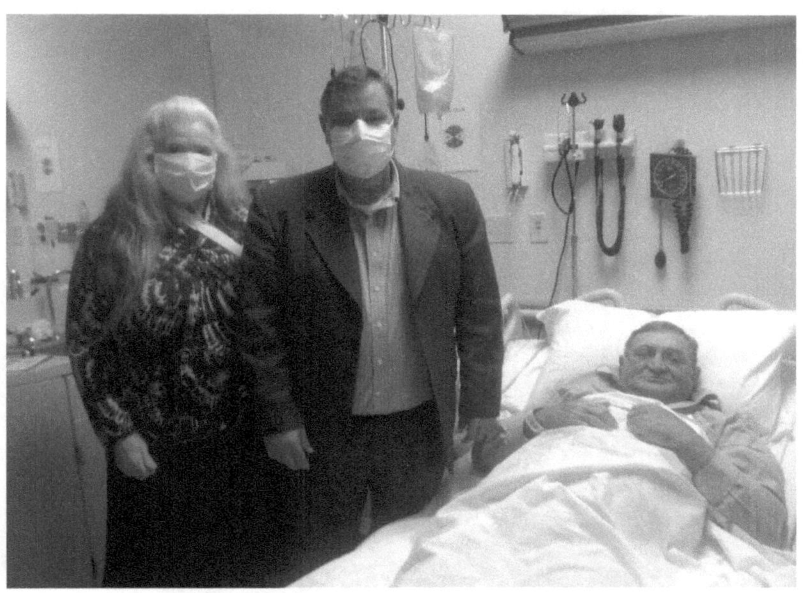

*Pastor Greg Roberts and his wife Faye who visited
and prayed with us at the hospital.*

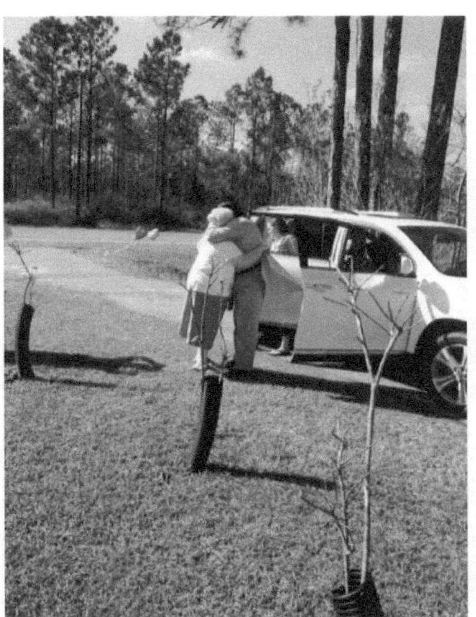

*I was so glad when I arrived home! We stopped the
vehicle so I could get out and hug my wife!*

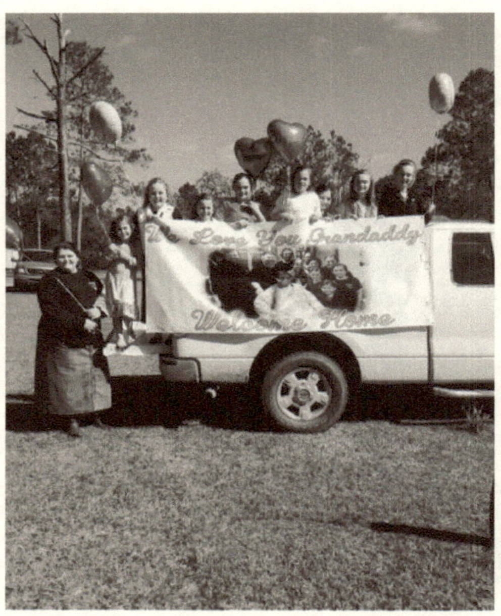

The welcoming party when I arrived home. They had
banners and balloons and lots of smiles.

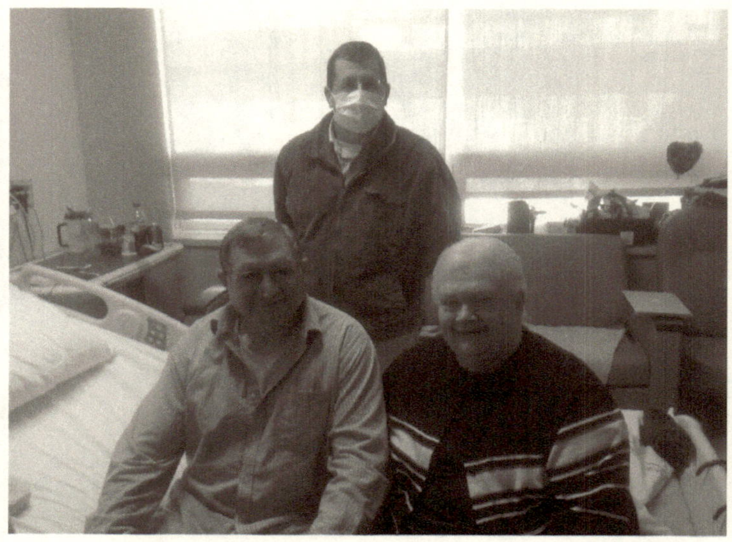

Pastor John Sewell visited me at Emory and served as interim pastor
for Pineview Holiness Baptist Church during my sickness.

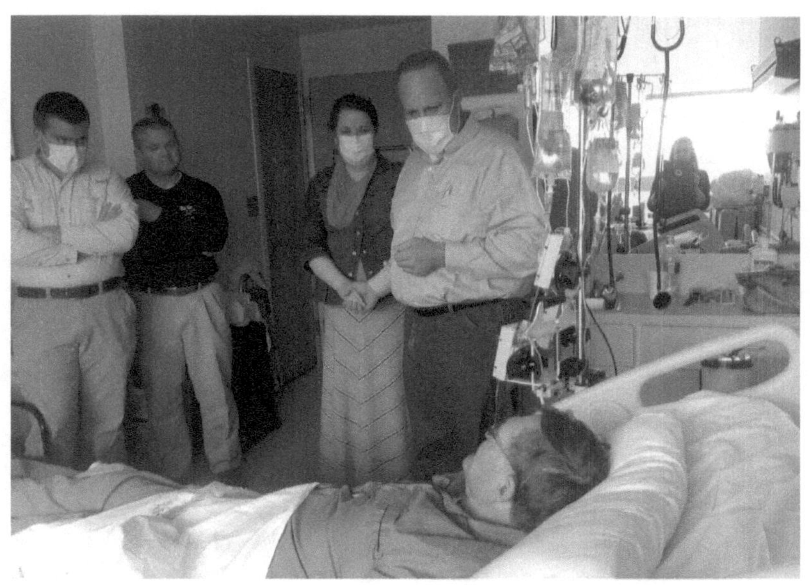

*Evangelist Nathan Johnson and his wife Jennifer brought encouraging words
and sang one of my special songs one afternoon that gave us great hope.*

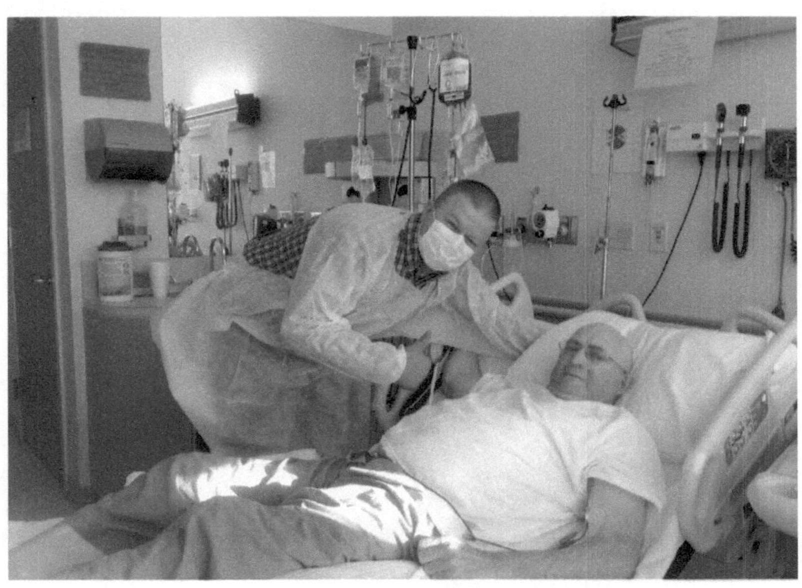

*Pastor Kyle Taft visited and brought a message
that strengthened our faith and hope.*

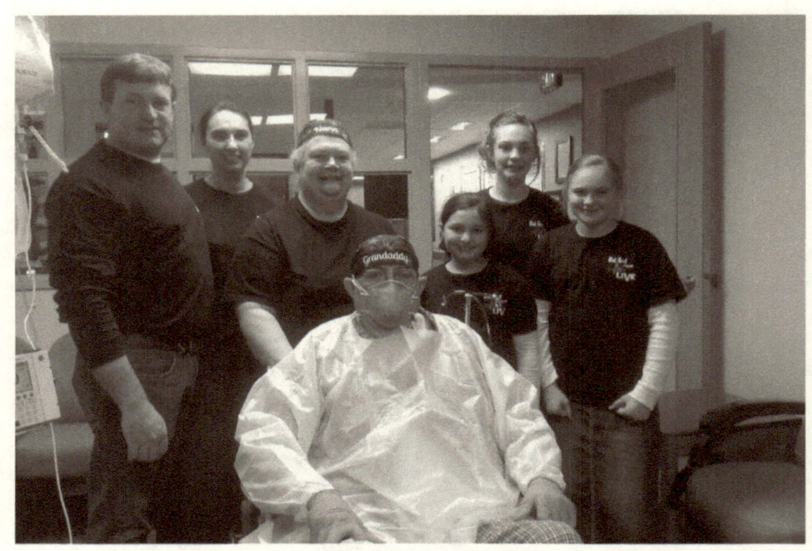

My son Mark and his family wearing their Ezekiel 16:6
shirts in support of our battle with AML.

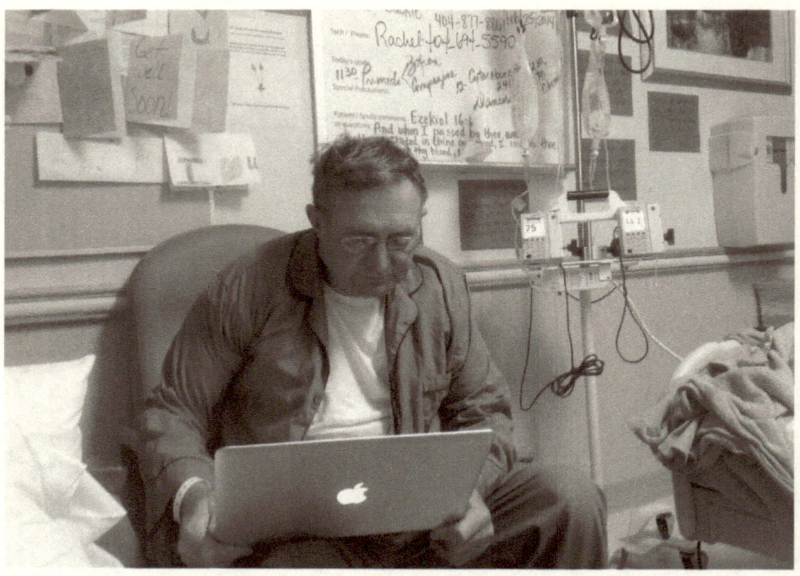

I really enjoyed reading the blog where friends sent encouraging messages.
Notice the faith-building Scriptures posted on the red construction paper
and written on the whiteboard. The birddog was still nearby.

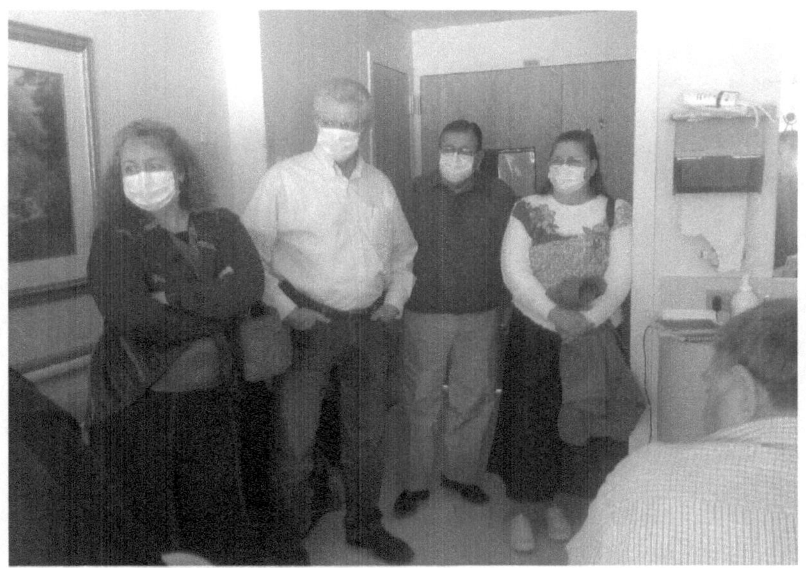

*Visitors from Pineview Holiness Baptist Church came
to check on their pastor and my family.*

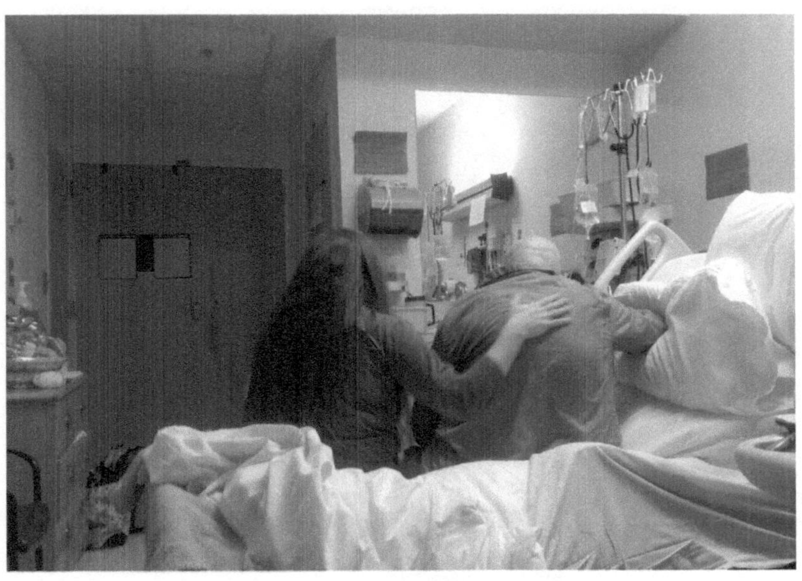

*My daughter Sherry praying for me while I was
fighting nausea, fever, and discomfort.*

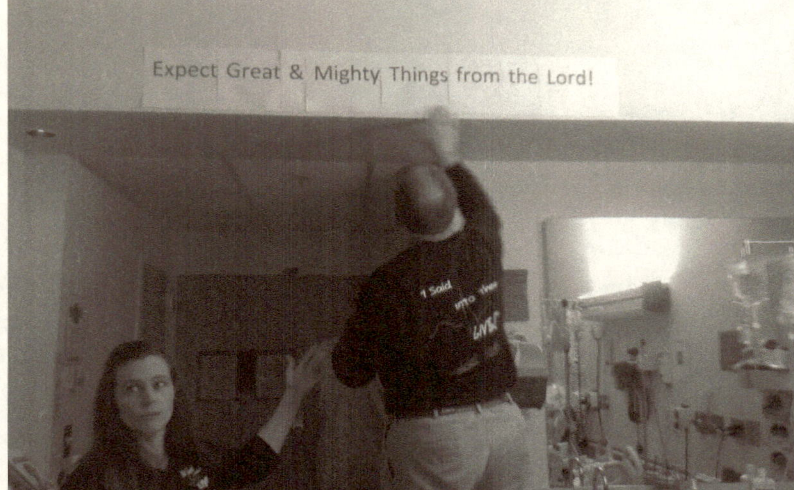

Sherry and her husband Silas (Doodlebug) posting encouraging words 'Expect great & mighty things from the Lord' where I could see them from my bed. We believe there is power in the Word.

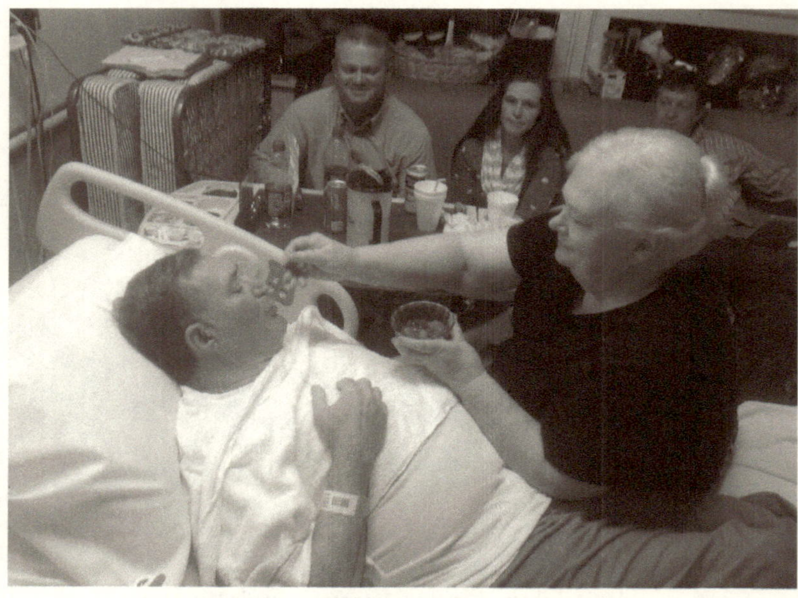

My wife Brenda feeding me during one of my sick times. Silas (Doodlebug) , Sherry, and Mark are watching the job well-done.

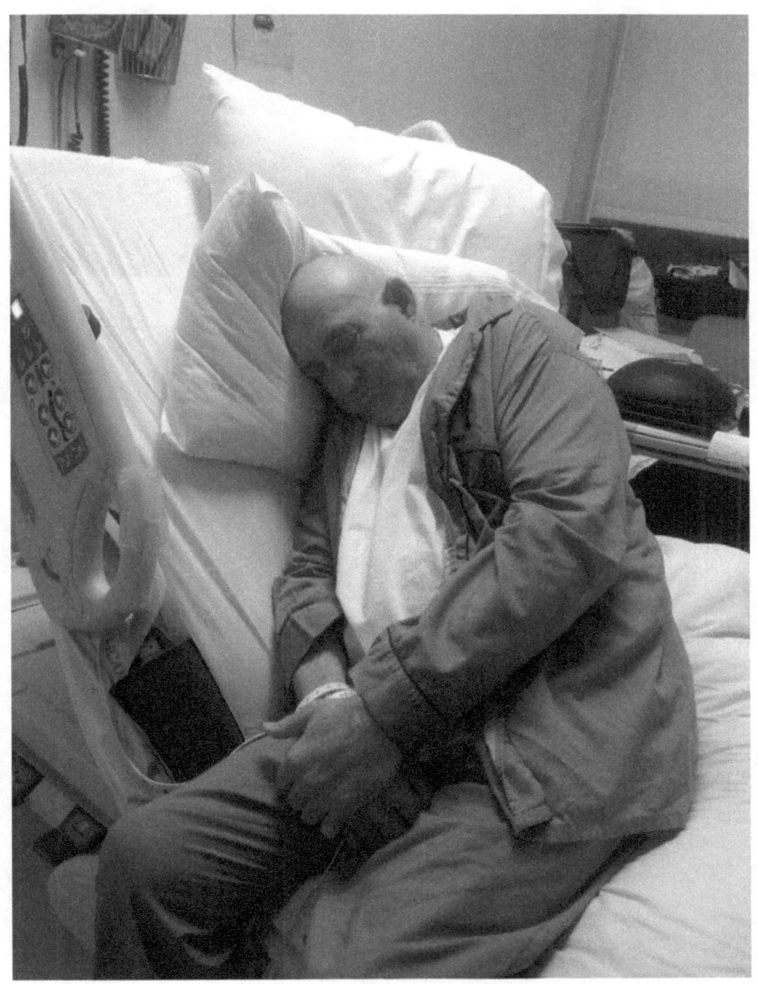

One of my sickest days. Hard to lay down and hard to sit up.

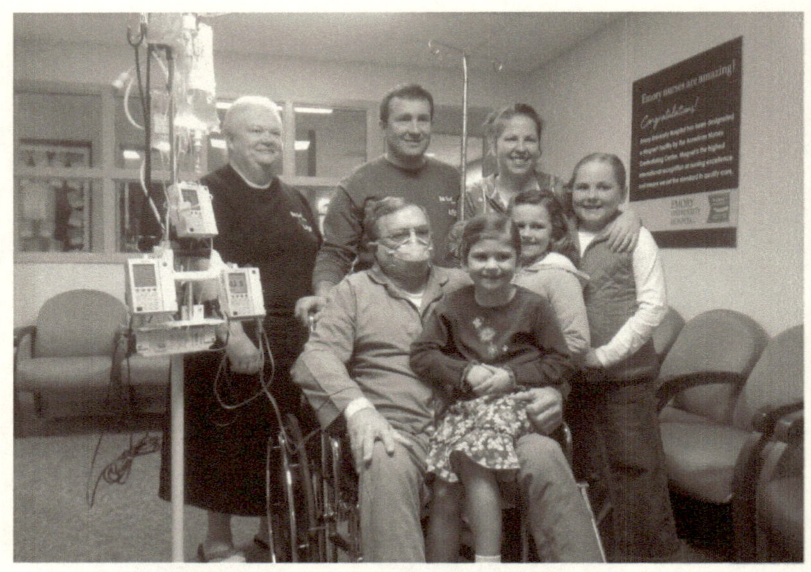

My son Terry and his family visiting with us in the waiting room. Still have the faithful birddog.

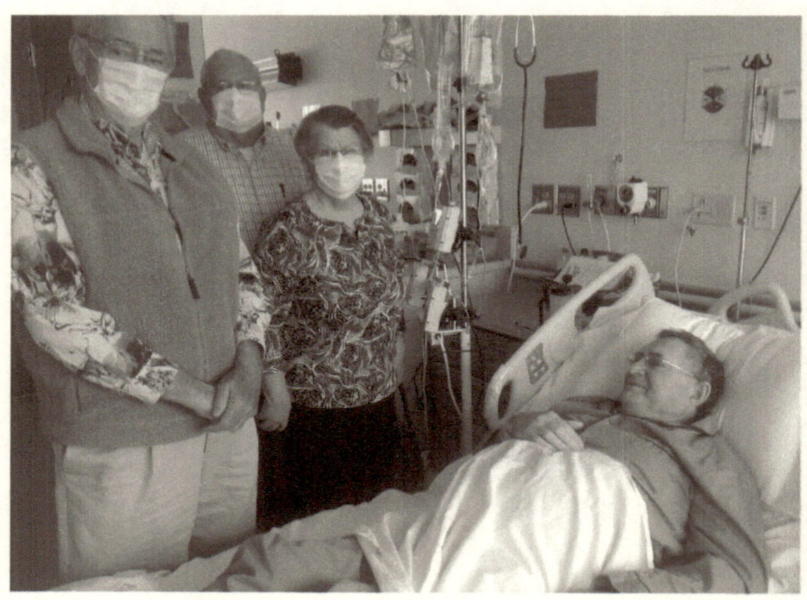

Evangelist & Missionary Neil Bridges, along with Bro. & Sis. Jimmy Bullard visiting and encouraging me in this great battle.

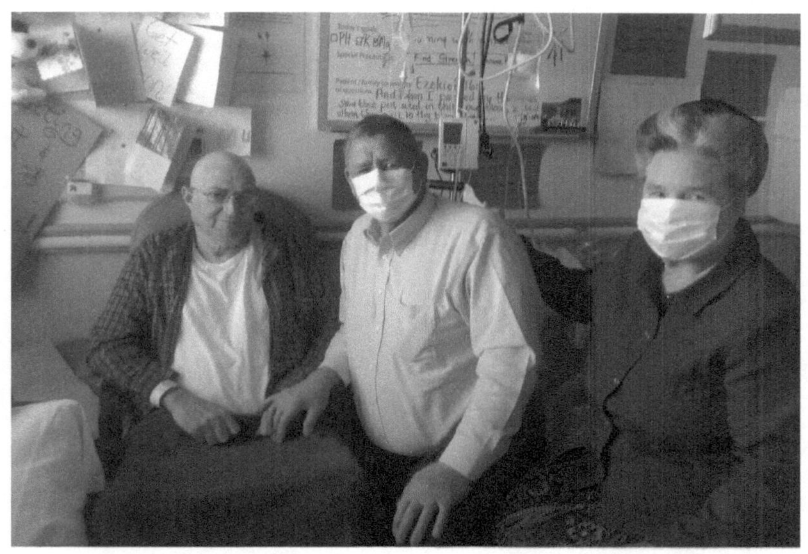

*Evangelist Larry Bowen and his wife Carolyn visited
us several times while we were at Emory.*

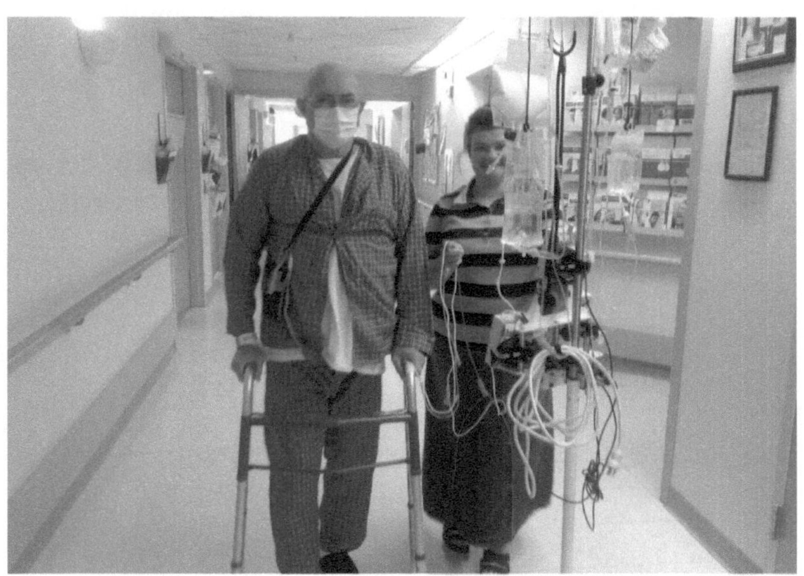

*Making a lap around the wing on E6. Some days it was a
struggle- notice all of the 'connections' that had to make the
trip outside of the room. The walker provided stability.*

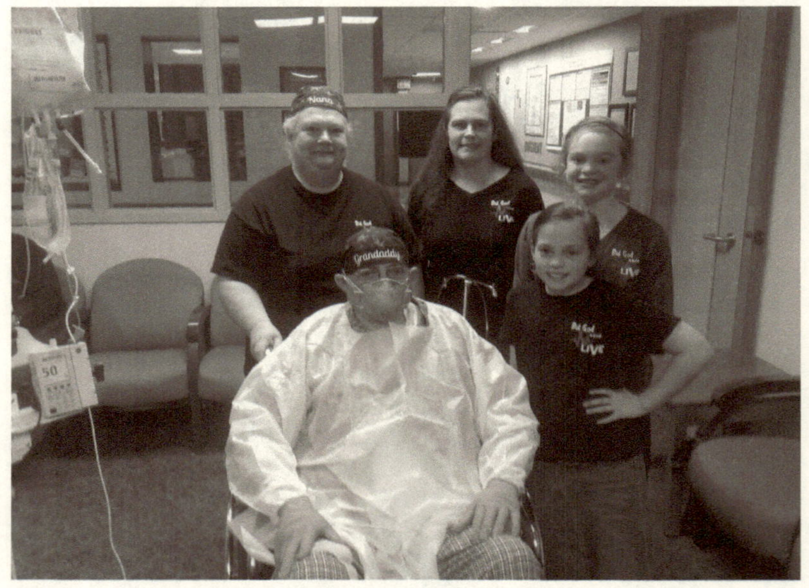

Immunity was almost nonexistent, so I had to suit up to visit the family.
Sherry and her girls are pictured here with their Ezekiel 16:6 shirts.

Additional pictures can be viewed on the blog
maintained during my sickness at
http://brothermorgan.weebly.com/photo-gallery.html